Sometimes the Dog is Smarter is an inspiring, fun, light-hearted and inf̶̶̶̶̶̶̶̶̶ ̶̶̶̶̶̶ ̶̶̶̶̶̶̶̶̶̶speaks to the incalculable benefits of literally having a companion walk through life with you and make the journey less stressful. Helpful for anyone who loves dogs, but especially for those looking to take the first step in training their very own service dog or Diabetes Alert Dog (DAD), it's a great go-to guide for getting started. Extensive resources to aid in a trainer's success are included. This book is also a must-read for anyone wanting more insight into the impact of living day-to-day with Type 1 diabetes!

Sofie Schunk, T1D since 2008, Co-Lead of the Diabetes Sports Project, Elite Athlete, MS Biomedical Engineering

Sometimes the Dog is Smarter is a wonderful journey from pet to partner. Kat takes us through the arduous process of training a Diabetes Alert Dog but this tale is so much more—truly an engaging love story between Abbey the DAD and her owner-trainer. It is extraordinary how much work and dedication it takes to train a DAD—illustrated through the author's vulnerability of revealing her diagnosis and ups and downs that everyone with diabetes goes through. The photographs that accompany each chapter brought me right into this well-written story filled with a dog's beautiful spirit, and the book left me wanting to meet Abbey and hear about more adventures with Abbey and Kat. Loved this book!

Virginia Valentine, APRN, BC-ADM, CDCES, FADCES, Clinica La Esperanza

This interesting book is about a dog trained by her owner to sense glycemic swings in blood glucose. The presence of these dogs is a wonderful asset because they can provide security in many ways, along with the gift of companionship. This story shows how Joslin Medalists and others are ingenious in their efforts to find ways that will allow them to live a regular life even when faced with Type 1 diabetes and its challenges.

George L. King, MD, Professor of Medicine and Ophthalmology, Harvard Medical School, and Chief Scientific Officer, Joslin Diabetes Center

Notes

This memoir is a true story and contains authentic names and photographs with the exception of a few individuals who requested privacy. In these cases, I have honored their wishes with the use of pseudonyms and a slight alteration of identifying details.

The terms Diabetes Alert Dog, Diabetic Alert Dog and DAD are used and often interchanged by people training, handling or working with clients. Within these fields of training and handling service dogs, the term Diabetic Alert Dog is still commonly found. In the medical field, the newer preferred term is Diabetes Alert Dog. The intent of the shift from "diabetic" to "diabetes" embraces an intentional stance upheld by many physicians, nurse educators and clinicians: that people living with diabetes are more than this disease, and that they should not, first and foremost, be labeled by their medical condition. Readers will find both terms used by different individuals represented within written passages and photographs that reflect their perspectives and training. The universal acronym of DAD stands for either: Diabetes Alert Dog or Diabetic Alert Dog; DAD and its plural—DADs—are terms used throughout these chapters.

Proceeds from the sales of this book will be donated, in part, to New Mexico's Camp 180° for children with diabetes and various United States-based diabetes programs that support building a better future for families.

TABLE OF CONTENTS

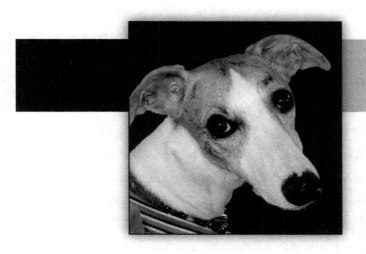

Chapter 1

Entry Into Another World

The idea strikes me as a bit on the crazy side: that I dare to think of training my beloved dog Abbey as a trusted companion to help me fight diabetes and plunging blood sugars. We have just retired from earning her championship on the show circuit, and though I miss my fellow handlers, I am so proud of this first-time accomplishment and all that has gone into it. While on the road, Abbey and I learned enough about each other to be in sync, and traveling together had made us even closer. When I gave up these special getaways once we finished the route to her championship, my heart ached. No doubt about it, this dog is unique. I crave being with her every day that I leave the house for my teaching job, or whenever I pursue hours of porcelain work in my weekly commitment to a local clay studio in a community of fellow artisans. Or everywhere, for that matter, I go without her.

So, what is the inspiration for thinking I'd actually be able to train a hound, of all breeds, as a trusted cohort in my fight to stay well despite living with Type 1? Perhaps the idea has been nurtured by the recent stream of articles on Diabetes/Diabetic Alert Dogs I've read in the last few years. Or, just as likely, realizing that Abbey is the most intelligent and wonderful whippet I have ever owned. I can't resist the pull of my revered dog's stare, with those baleful eyes exuding fervent pleas for more play, more challenges and never-ending affection. Guilt regularly singes my conscience when we are apart—that I'm not working with her enough; that she is bored at home and needs more cognitive stimulation than I am providing. Or, maybe, as my friend Sarah suggests, it is as simple as the fact that I thrive on setting up new challenges, and this endeavor is, in every sense of the word, a challenge to be mastered, just like the blessed but hard-earned triumph of ribboning at an agility or obedience trial or in the competitive show ring.

There is no doubting the lure—may my fellow lovers of the hound and mixed breed luring coursing world pardon the pun—and the impact of this kind of training. Or my need for it. The fact that I have not been hospitalized in years from plunging blood sugars is due to diligent testing and checking of my glucose level every few hours of every day. Using modern equipment and technology to inform me of these levels and when it's an acceptable time to eat has been crucial to my ability to live a relatively normal life. For now, let's not count the times I've been sidelined by equipment failure of these newer technologies. In other words, being in the right place at the right time with the right equipment, and learning how to use this information, has been my salvation.

And, strangely enough, so has luck. I've never been able to discount its role in helping me escape potential catastrophes that threaten to come crashing down; the ones that might undo my carefully orchestrated daily routine in the form of fainting or being carted off to a hospital in the throes of low blood sugar gone awry. I do everything possible to avoid coming to that. That is why, beyond my reliance on helpful equipment and a heap of hard-earned experience, luck, for me, is a somewhat mystical but humbly acknowledged force in my life. A bonus, of sorts. I'm thankful that I have learned to thwart most health-related catastrophes with a little luck. But I also realize that luck cannot be counted on in any way, shape or form to guide one's way through living well with diabetes.

Not every day runs smoothly when you live with this crazy up-and-down disease. There are many humbling episodes embedded in my memory bank, and I dread thinking of all the brain cells lost from a number of terrifying episodes that might have landed me in a hospital if help had not been nearby.

One particular summer spent as a young, new camper at Camp Firefly in Spring Mount, Pennsylvania illustrates the nuances of trying to achieve control when you are consistently grappling with exhausting fluctuations between higher-than-normal blood sugars and crashing lows. I spent six glorious years at this camp—a special place whose staff catered to children and young adults with Type 1. Once every year, for two entire weeks, I felt secure, treasured and connected; not singled out or different. It was like the most wonderful "opposite day" every day, where my camp friends and I rejoiced in diabetes being the norm. A heavenly feeling—except for the sweep of well-meaning residents and nurses trying to lower my sugar-drenched urine to a level as low as possible in the decades before daily home glucose testing and real-time blood sugar tracking with a Continuous Glucose Monitor (CGM). Trying to be a model diabetic and follow their advice, I consented to greatly increased amounts of syringe-delivered insulin doses which moved me, ashen and zombie-like, through my camp days while waves of crashing reactions upended my sense of control. Shaking, numbness around my mouth, legs and fingertips, an onslaught of sharp headaches brought on by an increase in recommended insulin dosage; all of it moved me dangerously out of control and unable to join in many activities. These close calls pushed me to realize that living so dangerously close to a constant low edge could prove catastrophic—despite the best of intentions by medical staff. I gained a new appreciation, early on, for the wisdom of bringing my glucose levels to as normal a range as possible, without being too high or too low, in what I realized was bound to be an uneven and difficult lifelong journey.

Yet another blood sugar near-disaster unnerved me as an adult although it wasn't an isolated incident. In the middle of coaching playwriting to my wonderfully clever, creative students, my blood sugar dropped violently and without warning. Home glucose monitoring was part of my routine by then, but the demands of being immersed "in the moment" while teaching those third, fourth and fifth graders typically won out over testing blood sugar levels as often as needed. Making time for taking proactive steps like having a snack was sometimes impossible in my role.

"Helen," I asked my co-teacher, "can you take over for a few?"

Helen glanced up at me from her stance while counting out algebra tiles with a few of the children. Her eyes widened. She didn't need to look twice to understand that I was in trouble.

"Sure," she said, not missing a beat. "Need to get something?"

4

I nodded, then stumbled to my desk and stirred my hand inside for something familiar. Candy, glucose tablets in a plastic tube, stale bagged and forgotten snacks, anything; I didn't care what showed up—just that it was there. My heart hammered loudly as my field of vision darkened. Helen deftly noticed my efforts and sent a trusted student to pry open a container of glucose tabs. I slumped into my chair, grateful that my colleague had my back and so ably covered our shared students. It took six tablets, a can of juice and twenty minutes to recover from the daze of my plunging blood sugar. This was more time than normally needed to be up again and running, but after that, like usual, I was miraculously "back." Helen didn't know it, and I chose not to reveal, how close I'd been to declaring an all-out emergency, nearly ready to surrender to calling 9-1-1.

Several years ago, I thought my luck had finally run out, having awakened from a never-ending dream at 5:00 a.m. with my heart pounding like a trapped bird. Not wanting to rouse my exhausted husband, I decided to take care of things myself by rolling from the warm covers and pulling myself along the walls into the master bathroom. Once there, I fell heavily on the commode and placed a chalky glucose tablet (they're seemingly stashed everywhere) into my mouth as my peripheral vision faded. At that point, my head rested on my lap.

Breathe deeply. But it was too late. I passed out onto the porcelain floor, enfolded in a black fog, my forehead slamming onto the metal toilet paper holder and trash can rim at my feet. The crash jarred my husband from the last of his sleep, and he came running at the hammering sounds falling like gigantic dominoes come to life.

He shoved yet another saving tablet into my mouth.

"No!" I moaned. "Don't want any. Go 'way.

A flash of clarity and a sense of panic helped me recall an early morning meeting I'd arranged to attend.

"Need to… get to work."

I was so far gone that the mashed-up glucose dribbled out in angry rejections. Despite my reaction, he stroked my hair and tried persuading me to suck on more tablets. My heart thumped as I lay on the hard floor like an ensnared roadrunner, thinking about time ticking by. One thing was certain: I knew I'd be late to that meeting with my colleagues.

When the most severe shaking finally subsided, I stood up, held onto the bathroom counter and blanketed my badly bruised face with an unusually heavy layer of makeup. All while muttering a few choice words at my lack of luck this time around and the extra attention I'd be sure to garner from colleagues.

Upon my arrival at work, I offered a lame excuse for my tardiness and was shocked that my comrades accepted it unconditionally. Didn't they know the truth? Couldn't they tell I was lying? Yet no one seemed troubled. It seemed only I carried the residue of guilt and shame.

This one was a close call with the effects of fuzzy thinking and my sluggish body lasting nearly a month. That this single episode could have such an impact scared me. Who knew what the effects were that couldn't be felt? Unanswerable questions stirred in my head: What if …someone doesn't hand me that glucose tablet or can of soda or orange juice? What if… my blood sugar drops when I'm driving and I don't sense it or there's no safe place to pull over? What if… I'm alone, in dire straits and can't manage to get what's needed? I've asked all these questions and more. My inability to come up with answers that cover these contingencies compelled me to cook up another plan.

This dilemma leads to a reluctant compromise: my agreement to try a newer technology called a Continuous Glucose Monitor. But I discover that using this tool to inform me about my diabetes management, while a godsend, is not without problems. For one, it takes an hour or more to calibrate after insertion. And two, I don't always wake when it beeps insistently, trying to warn me that low blood sugar is at hand.

Despite my blood sugars stabilizing better by using a CGM, there are still glitches in trying to manage my diabetes as well as my physicians and I would like. Inconsistencies in the timing of my daily activities like yoga, dog agility classes, walking, or gardening, and an overreliance on my insulin pump's insulin-to-carb ratios play a role and demand more active intervention on my part so that diabetes does not control me as much as it has. I know something else is still needed if I dare to believe that my life, in spite of diabetes, can be better. But what is it that I've not yet considered?

One night, cuddled up on the sofa amid a harem of sleepy dogs, I look at sweet Abbey and am lost in thought and possibility. How can my dog's intense connection with me and her love of people work to my advantage?

My mind races at the chance to be even more proactive about living with diabetes and to find a way to keep my cherished dog with me more often. I am open to nearly anything that could make a difference in my life. It is at this turning point on a late New Mexico's summer evening filled with the trill of desert cicadas, I do what any reasonable, rational person in slippers, poised on the brink of willingness to combine luck and reality, would do: I Google service dogs and diabetes.

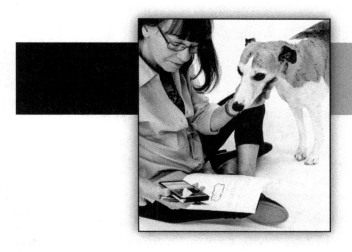

Chapter 2

Can We Do This? DAD Or DUD?

This is my story of reckoning—the day I finally come to terms with making a logical decision on what it takes to live my best life. It marks the start of new understandings about living with diabetes and a readiness, after more than forty decades of living with Type 1, to tackle choices that will forever change me. Little do I understand the true implications of my choices, but still, I move forward.

The more I search online about Diabetic Alert Dogs, the more my curiosity soars. There are several reputable groups listed in New Mexico and elsewhere: Assistance Dogs of the West (ADW); the Animal Humane Association; Service Dogs of New Mexico; local trainers offering classes for service dog training and scent classes. The possibility of purchasing a ready-trained Diabetic Alert Dog is out there, too. But all of these choices seem like lengthy, pricy propositions. And then an epiphany jolts me; the self-doubt and excuses are no answer at all. Aren't

I willing to commit to the hard road ahead if it can make my life better? This well-deserved chiding finally gains enough steam to move me forward.

I contact Arie Deller by email—a dog trainer recommended by my trusted agility instructor Hannah Agee, who seems to know everyone worth knowing in the dog world—asking if she is up to the task. What does she think about the wisdom, or folly, of training a sighthound to detect smells signifying low blood sugar?

By now, the little information I've kludged together on the Internet makes it clear that the best service dogs make great use of their noses, have unflappable temperaments and one other little thing—they should not be too distractible. The irony of my proposal to train a hound, whose breeds are often generalized as somewhat inattentive and aloof, doesn't escape me. This didn't hold true for most of my whippet family over the years, but I hope this trainer might overlook these common breed stereotypes. I hold my breath and wonder if the request is too audacious to even suggest.

Arie's response is cautious, but open, as she bombards me with questions:

Hi Kat. Can you tell me why you want a service dog?

Why don't you just travel to Santa Fe for regular service dog and Diabetic Alert Dog training with an existing group that's known for their work?

What traits does your dog have that make you think she's capable of doing this work?

> And what can you tell me about your diabetes—how do you handle high and low blood sugars?

Excited now, I answer her questions as fast as she shoots them to me, as honestly as possible—except for one bias, and a big one at that.

My fingers fly over the keys in my quest to describe my dog's positive traits:

> I swear my dog is a genius—for a whippet, that is. She's the smartest, calmest dog I've ever owned, and so tuned in to me and other people! We're an amazing team, and that's what I'm banking on to do this kind of training. I think she can do this. Can you help us?

I want to convince her and hope she'll be persuaded by what I have to say. But the initial test is yet to come, and I pray that I won't be proven wrong. A few days pass before Arie's reply comes.

> Hey, Kat. It's worth looking at. Let's meet and we can talk more about it. I'd like to see Abbey for myself and figure out what we can do.

With that, I commit to a consultation with a relative stranger that leaves everything I hope for up in the air. Three weeks of waiting, wondering, wishing. Twenty-one days of working to reinforce novice obedience commands with Abbey. Over five hundred hours of trying to objectively observe and assess if my sweet sighthound can pass muster in the most basic step on this long journey.

My hopes are far too big to corral into this first meeting. My emotions rise and fall like oncoming electrical summer storms in the Land of Enchantment. One time span crashes into another as D-Day, circled in red on the calendar, looms, and I pretend not to count the days.

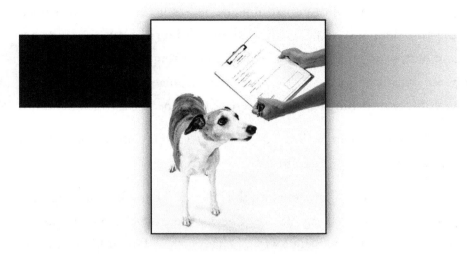

Chapter 3

First Appraisal

D-day, also scribbled in bright red marker as DAD Day on the family calendar, blows in the first week of February; the 7th to be exact. I had spent much of the previous month reminding myself, over and over, to lower my expectations. Right now, they are hopes and pipe dreams. I know it is crucial to be open to any words of wisdom Arie shares about what it really takes to train a service dog. And it remains to be seen whether she is willing, or even the right person, to be my accomplice in training.

A few minutes before Arie's scheduled arrival at my house, I place my other two dogs outside in their kenneled yard. Distractions, for both Abbey and me, are something to be avoided at all costs.

When the doorbell rings, I welcome Arie while gripping hard on Abbey's collar. Standing at the door is a smiling woman with short, chopped, red-toned hair, tattoos and two small lip rings. She is much younger than me but looks strong and self-assured. I like that. I open the glass door and, to her credit, she doesn't flinch as my dog sniffs her and jumps up, hound-style, in exuberant greeting. I, on the other hand, visibly shrink at my canine's lack of manners; her greeting is entirely my fault for not teaching her how to behave when people arrive at my door.

"Come in, you must be Arie," I say, "and this is Gabby-Abbey. She'll take a minute or two to calm down."

She nods and follows me into the kitchen. Thankfully, my precious girl quickly settles alongside me. Phew. I imagine the trainer already making her first impressions while I chatter away. For all I know, we've been scored as possible successes or potential failures from the moment she arrived. Trying to counter my dog's uninhibited greeting, I give Abbey a few quick commands to demonstrate that she can follow them: "turn right", "turn left," "drop." I don't know if this wins us any points, but I fervently hope so.

"Good to see she understands those," Arie says.

I exhale slowly, glad she'd caught this action.

"If it's okay, I'd like to spend most of our time today talking about what you want," Arie says. "And get a feel for whether Abbey can be trained as a service animal. Look at how we might be able to work together."

"Yes," I reply. "That's what I thought you'd want to do."

In all truthfulness, I don't know one iota about what might unfold. I am as naïve as a newborn pup about service dog training. But that leaves me open to considering all kinds of possibilities.

Arie opens her notebook. Pen poised, she takes copious notes as I answer her questions. Impressive, I think, the amount of detail she so meticulously records.

Arie asks about my diabetes; how I handle it and what glucose levels I can physically perceive. Do I feel all, most or none of my dropping blood sugars? The intense focus on me and my diabetes skews what I really thought she'd most want to do at this appointment—assess my dog—and it forces me to concentrate on giving her the background information she needs.

Arie's questions also push me to reflect on how I feel about sharing the most important and intimate essentials related to controlling my diabetes and the ways I handle challenges. I appreciate her attempt to grasp what my everyday life and needs are, especially in the context of the huge task I want to undertake.

As a neophyte, I realize how essential it is to have a trainer's assistance. Just starting on this long and unfamiliar road of service dog training places me in unfamiliar territory, and if there is any hope to accomplish the required tasks, a partnership of some sort is the next step.

Several notebook pages and forty minutes later, Arie looks up. "Well," she says, "I can see that you have enough background to work with Abbey between the times we'd meet. And I think Abbey has a nice temperament. It's obvious she is close to you. It's worth trying to train her if you're willing to do the work."

"Really?" I ask. Her pronouncement that I can proceed with training leaves me dumbstruck. No real formal assessment beyond the checklist she holds in her hands? No need to test my dog? I am surprised, but how keen the quiet, but substantial, observational powers of a good trainer are!

"Yes," Arie replies. "We'll need to figure out what blood sugar readings you want her to react to so she can signal you."

I have to consider one issue in particular, knowing the importance of this choice. Most people train their DADs to signal for both highs and lows, but for me, this would mean no peace at all most days. My Type 1 life has always been like this: waking up low and having my blood sugar rebound in response and then trying to treat the highs with more insulin, only to sometimes repeat the low-high cycle several times a day. Isn't being on that rollercoaster what most Type 1s experience? I know better, of course, but for someone with more "brittle" or labile diabetes, a past label some nurses and doctors have used on me, it makes the quest for stabilizing blood sugars a constant goal.

I follow my inclination and ask, "Can we just work on having Abbey learn to signal me for low blood sugar? At least to start?"

I describe how training Abbey to signal for both lows and highs might never give either of us a moment's rest.

"Low blood sugar is the most serious thing that can happen to me. I could end up in the emergency room if I don't keep track of when my sugars fall." What I really need most is some way for her to tell me when my blood sugar is dropping. Not as much when my blood sugar is high."

Arie nods. "Sounds like a good idea," she replies. "Let's start by training Abbey to signal you for low blood sugar. We can always add a high glucose alert later."

Part of me wonders if Arie accepts my goal because she thinks the job might be simpler to train a hound, versus a more standard breed of service dog like Labradors or Golden retrievers, to alert to just one issue. Or does she truly support the wisdom of narrowing our target goal? I can't tell.

"What number, say, would you want to work with?" she adds.

I nod and reflect on the question: what reading on my home meter or Continuous Glucose Monitor would indicate that I am plummeting into a danger zone and need to treat myself with juice, candy, glucose or a snack in order to be okay?

"Probably around 55, maybe 60," I reason. "At a reading of 65 or 70, I am still 'safe.'" No huge emergency. I can test and eat a snack, and things are usually fine. But at 55 or even 63, it means my blood sugar is on the way down and something needs to be done quickly."

"Sounds good," she says. "We'll need to work on training Abbey on public access behaviors, too. They're very important. Before our next meeting, I want you to do two things."

I scribble down the name of the Diabetic Alert Dog training manual she recommends, noting to order it on Amazon and delve into it when it arrives. Thankfully, it sounds short and to the point.

Arie notes, "As you read the book, think carefully about the work involved in training a service dog and if you really want to do it. It's a huge commitment and not such a simple thing."

"I will," I assure her.

The second task seems both simple and complex. That's because I can't help but take this part of her request personally.

"Make a list of all the words and commands Abbey knows. Ones she understands," she instructs.

I nod, happy at the chance to do this. I have compiled these lists before for many of our dogs. It's a fun check on what we've taught them.

Arie adds, "And the percentage of times she completely follows through on those words and commands, showing how much she understands them."

What?! A warning bell chimes in my brain. Danger! Danger! Her words strike fear in my heart; set me shivering with unease. Understanding? Percentage? Yet another caveat for having my dog pass muster?

I wonder if Abbey's level of knowledge and follow-through is even measurable. Not so sure about this and asking myself if this first mountain can be climbed, I pray all my foolish boasting about my dog's extraordinary level of intelligence—for a whippet—isn't going to come back to haunt me.

Arie and I set up our next appointment for the following month. Certainly, this is time enough to tackle my new to-do list and brush up on consistency—my dog's and my own. With this goal in mind, as soon as she departs, I head out, said special beast in tow, to refill the doggie treat jar. I somehow suspect that a hefty supply of these tasty morsels will be a persuasive and much-needed ally in the weeks ahead.

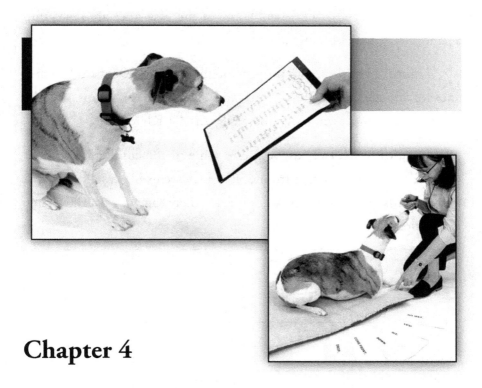

Chapter 4

More Than Words Can Say

New obligations at work force me to postpone the next session with Arie. We would now be meeting, not four, but six long weeks after our initial session. I am disappointed but focus on moving forward.

To keep my mind off the lengthy span between training sessions, I tackle the first thing Arie has asked me to do: my husband Bob and I compile a list of vocabulary we think Abbey knows well. It gets trickier as I find that we both want extra credit for every word we've ever shared with her! That's how competitive we are when the going gets tough and we have to be accountable.

"Bob, what about the agility words she already knows?"

"Yep," he replies. "Let's see. Some of the easy ones are tap, jump and weave. What else can you come up with?"

"Hmm," I reply, envisioning one of our training sessions. "Touch is another one she understands. 'Wait' and 'stay' when she jumps onto the box for the countdown, remember? Oh, and 'watch me.'

We howl hysterically as we mime some of the commands to each other. The list that emerges from our first try seems like a solid one, but more words are added as we observe them at play during daily interactions:

come	sit	drop	toy
down	wait	touch	bad
tap	watch me	ball	good girl!
toy	go right	go left	crate
weave	jump	stay	treat
walk	breakfast	dinner	open
bingo	walk it	go	chair
teeter	tunnel	okay	bed
give	water	tire	up
Mommy	Daddy	Pop Pop	off
heel	stand	pee-pee	agility
out	kiss	catch	water

Flipping the paper over, we add others we've missed recording:

cheese	under	Tess	Zoe
gentle	Get the ___	Get it!	speak
give	chute	tunnel	bunny car
stop	bath	more	Stop

shower	stand	mas	come
front	shhh!	shake	Gimme five!
High five!	Daddy treat	Tally ho!	

The rest of the page remains blank as the two of us dutifully struggle to recall any additions, but we strike out. All types of words, especially those related to basic obedience, are on the initial list. Others are pure fun. In all, well over seventy make the cut. The list isn't too meager for a young sighthound just under two years of age. Pouring over the page in front of me, I mull whether Arie wants to assess my dog's intelligence or identify words from the list that might be useful for scent training to signal falling blood sugars.

Then I tackle the task that has set so much pressure squarely on my shoulders: how often, or what percentage of the time, does my dog follow and understand each word? Hmmm. Good question. I try considering words and commands that she discerns through the things she loves to do without hesitation, and this seems to help boost the size of our word list enough to make me happier. Maybe even the tiniest bit smug.

That feeling quickly vanishes as I delve into the task. The light that Arie must have hoped I'd see is beginning to shine, as I review words that my dog follows nearly one hundred percent of the time. Are they the ones we'll use to train her? I'm not certain, but just in case, I highlight the top ten or so words: Go. Wait. Touch. Tap. Drop. Stay. High five. The others, glaring naked from the sheet, speak volumes about the need for more training. But I am encouraged and wonder if I will need to choose one "power word" to use in our DAD training. I don't really know, but with my path now more clearly lit, Abbey and I work our tails off—both canine and human—at sticking these words to memory.

While vocabulary and follow-through fill my time with several training sessions each day, the DAD training book I had ordered finally arrives. I reserve an hour to tackle the first chapter of Training Your Diabetic Alert Dog by Rita Martinez and Susan Barns, which focuses on the problematic trait of distractibility. Uh oh, not again. The authors must have been thinking of hounds' distractibility when they wrote this. Like an arrowhead notching my heart, the first section quickly undermines the initial confidence I'd righteously placed in my DAD goal. Not because of its tone, which is friendly and helpful, but because of my own vulnerabilities. Up and down my hopes seem to roll, and where they'll stop, I surely don't know.

The next day brings a rekindling of surging determination, and I voraciously tackle training with the most powerful weapon I have on hand. And such an ironic weapon it is since, as a person with diabetes, my life is so necessarily fixated, day in and day out, on food. That's right. Chow. Grub. Sustenance. Call it what you will. But this is just not any food; oh no! This is apparently a "'super food'"—announced right on the package in bold black lettering as "'healthy and nutritious.'" Truly, I am not sure if I care one whit if it is nutritious or not. It only needs to be delicious enough to help connect Abbey's neurons to actions, just as liver bait pieces had worked their persuasive magic in New Mexico, Colorado and Arizona conformation rings. This is how my dog and I find ourselves immersed in something that approaches a food-throwing marathon designed to reward desired training behaviors.

"Touch," I tell her. Abbey gently pushes her wet, pointy nose into the palm of my right hand. A morsel of gooey salmon lays ready as an immediate reward.

"YES!" I say. Then, "Tap." Tap is a recall command used on the agility field; one she knows. The light bulb above her head seemingly hums.

Pushing Abbey just like I challenge my human students to think flexibly, I give her a few different words, or synonyms, for similar behaviors. I want her to recognize that some of these words mean the same thing and she should give me the same behavior for them. I use these over and over, waiting for that light bulb to show me that she understands what I am asking of her.

"Tap," I tell her.

"Good girl, tap." I toss a small treat.

"Touch," I say.

Abbey looks at me, hesitates for a moment, and tap-touches my hand.

My heart soars at Abbey's successes. She understands. Again and again, treats are readily given for these consistent responses. I feel like a miracle worker as salmon flows freely, sometimes dropping onto the tiled kitchen floor or falling onto counters. That is no problem, either: All three of my dogs volunteer to snarf up and perform for every shred whose scent permeates the air.

"If I was a salmon," I tell my husband, wriggling right and left to prove my point, "that dog would come running no matter what request came out of my mouth. She'd pay attention to everything I asked."

"No doubt," he replies. I hope that isn't mocking disbelief I hear dripping from his voice. His smile, though, gives him away.

Inwardly, I bless the helpfulness of our nearby Costco for this treasured behavior-shaper. Outwardly, I coax and faithfully work with Abbey day and night, giving commands and enough enthusiastic yeses to uplift dour crowds. It is most definitely the manna of heaven for food-driven dogs, and mine is one happy animal performing for any bits I throw her way. As a trainer, I am immensely pleased, too, getting to regularly lick a fork filled with such nutritious and delicious carb-free leftovers.

The salmon-filled sessions continue day after yummy day with fine results, although my hands stink mightily, much like autumn's pungent, bursting scent of yellow-flowered desert chamisa. My friend Victoria in Santa Fe thinks this is hilarious, advising that my chances for such a coup most obviously depend on bottling "Eau de Salmon." I get it. I just hope we aren't swimming up a creek.

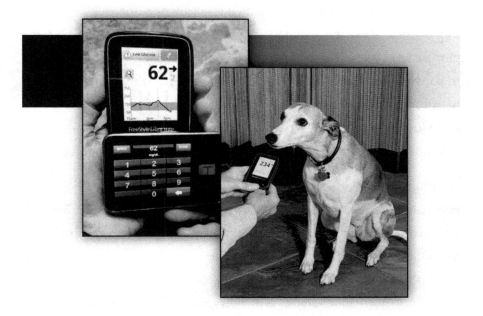

Chapter 5

Personal Choices

Everyone has to make choices that work for them, and in the scheme of coming up with a plan to train Abbey as a DAD, I end up making two important decisions. One is common sense, and the other is less conforming to normal DAD-training based on my personal needs and lifestyle.

Figuring out which problem to address and put at the very top of my DAD training decisions is easy, since it is the central issue faced by nearly everyone impacted by this disease: falling blood sugar. Its stealthy habit of pouncing in unexpected places makes its impact problematic, at best. This is the culprit that makes smooth sailing through each day something those of us with diabetes can't take for granted.

I am often confronted with this challenge, particularly upon awakening, when less attuned to physical and mental signs that my glucose level is low. It has crossed me countless times while I've engaged in conversations with friends and colleagues. And when I am immersed in specific tasks, the physical signals coursing through my body and brain are too-easily rendered mute or undetectable—even in the face of having available, informative data from my now often-worn CGM.

Plummeting glucose incidents during social interactions are particularly challenging due to how self-conscious they make me feel. Granted, this is a topic in and of itself, and one I've grappled with all my life. When they occur, my brain tries to circumvent the impact of these plunges by sweet-talking me with its "I won't let anyone see that you're not normal" charade. Not everyone feels such a deep sense of mortification, but the sheer sense of surprise I feel at being "unmasked" in public can be terrifying.

I've come to call my brain's manner of dealing with these plunges the "Triple D" defense—deny, deny, deny (at all cost) that anything is wrong. Suddenly caught by gaps in its own reasoning, my ego-driven brain belatedly bows in a moment of defeat. 'Raise that flag of surrender!' it screams, as my heart pounds, my ears ring and my ability to speak in coherent sentences vanishes.

When this happens, I sheepishly realize it is often too late to avoid embarrassment, and stepping out of the social game is imperative. There is no leeway to "cover up" some of these steep plunges. These are the incidents that shake my emotions and core sense of self. The times when I feel shocked to catch my own voice—as if hearing it from another dimension—attempting a sweet apology, excusing myself from conversation, and turning away to a place of temporary refuge. One where I can finally suck in the carbs that my body demands in order to safely recover and reclaim a new normal. Relief comes—but at a price.

I make a firm commitment to train Abbey to alert me to dropping glucose levels. It's an obvious first choice and a wise one to keep me from tripping through the shaky realm of being called on social miscues or my fear of going past the point of no return by passing out from a rapid, all-encompassing low. It's mighty convenient that I can envision my angel of rescue coming to me in a furry, adoring form.

I consider what other things my wonderful canine might do to support me and end up brainstorming a list of situations that will drive a meaningful DAD-training plan. Mantras swirl in my head, allowing me to ponder what was, what is, and what could be. Soon, details and pictures spill forth and I scribble them onto a tablet. Then they make their way to my fingers hammering ideas on a keyboard. Immersed in deep reflection, I give myself permission to grapple with, and name, many of these real, honest issues about living and struggling with diabetes—ones that have tapped anger, hope and even denial in me.

When I finally stop writing, the resulting document provides me with a sense of personal clarity. The most obvious one jumps out at me, confirming my earliest inclination about working on a backup warning system—my dog—for letting me know about low blood sugar episodes. Nothing else is more critical, and it's so important a commitment that I begin panicking as I realize the immense weight of my obligation to successfully train Abbey. Having read many layperson-oriented articles and journal studies about DADs, as well as talking with DAD owner-handlers, I know enough to clearly understand the importance of getting clear and consistent alerts from my dog. She will need to be trained as my backup system to any cues I miss—the ones that typically happen within my working environment. And although I strive to keep crashing "lows" from impacting my work world, they sometimes do.

After thinking about this and taking a few deep breaths, I add notes to indicate some of the 'wishes' worth holding onto for future training and assistance from my dog.

My DAD could be trained to help with:

1- Warning me about dropping/low blood sugar

2- high blood sugar

3- rising blood sugar levels (how will she know this?)

4- carrying an emergency id for me

5- carrying emergency contact info

6- helping me access candy or glucose tabs? Maybe by having some kind of pocket or a vest that holds these?

7- ? Can a DAD be trained to alert to the smell of ketones?

8- Finding me sugar/glucose when I need it!

Getting help if I need it … HOW?

Although not on this list, I spend a few minutes contemplating the CGM that I'm destined to use more frequently until it becomes part of my diabetes management routine. In the past, there have been times both my CGM and insulin pump have failed to provide me with enough solid data on which I base insulin dosing and carbohydrate intake decisions. These challenges have arisen primarily when my CGM is in calibration mode (where no tracking of blood sugar levels is available for up to two hours) and times that my CGM-pump combination give suspect readings that don't match how I am feeling. These issues already let me know that I'll continue to depend on Abbey as a backup tool and source of information. The ups and downs of this disease don't always abide by my rules or expectations. I realize, too, the need to make time to thoroughly understand the role of using a CGM and its data in tandem with my dog's alerts to any low glucose levels.

After establishing these first training decisions, I tackle what should come after training Abbey for the behaviors that alert me to "lows." And once trained and mastered, what do I need to consider for training my dog to do at a later time?

Again, I refocus on the list and add more stars to these secondary ideas, reaching a crucial point where a personal and potentially controversial decision has to be made: what to do about training my DAD to alert to high blood sugar. And surprisingly, I decide to let it be; to do nothing. That's right.

Some might question the wisdom of excluding a high blood sugar alert from DAD behavior-training, because it is a huge challenge faced by Type 1s—no matter their age. Particularly for families of children and teens, as well as those with unstable glucose levels, this is a vital issue. In general, training a DAD to alert to both "highs" and "lows" outside the normal range is an important consideration for anyone facing diabetes.

I make a mental note to talk with my endocrinology team about my health issues and seek the opinion of my mentor Arie and then push myself to review them thoroughly. Over time, I stick with my original analysis: to train Abbey to only alert for low glucose levels. What persuades me? These personal facts: daily multiple testing of my blood sugars; CGM use; accessible on-hand supplies to diagnose and proactively treat high glucose; and deep awareness of the physical sensations that accompany these high blood sugar levels. During my years as a pre-teen, teen and in college, dog alerts to both glucose extremes would have been essential. How I wish, now, that I had had the support of a DAD in those days; a trained dog as a teammate who could have helped prevent several of my hospitalizations and struggles. But after deep reflection and throwing every possible question at the wisdom of bucking the norm, I am surprisingly confident that "not now" is the right decision. Even so, though training my dog to alert to high blood sugars does not appear to be a critical life-or-death matter for me, it will deservedly stay on my radar and await future consideration.

Another factor plays into my decision to let go of additional alert training for these "highs": concern for my dog's mental and physical health. To examine my actual needs and their consequences, I review my blood sugar history over the past weeks, months and then years on end. With these data in hand, I consider what everyday life might be like for my DAD if she had to constantly alert me to both lows and highs, as happens with rebounding glucose levels—high sugars dropped too low by dosing extra insulin in a day-long impact—that I tackle a few times most weeks. I shake my head trying to visualize this scenario: no rest for my dog, and no breaks for me! Bound to drive both of us bonkers. Having Abbey carry this level of responsibility 24/7 with my lifelong pattern of rebounding blood sugars seems like an unrealistic expectation. It's a dilemma, for certain, with no clear outcomes to let me know if I am making the right decision, but an important consideration that must be based on one's personal needs.

Focusing on Abbey by making us equal partners and finding satisfaction and joy in working together is key. Everything I plan for training my dog must account for our personal strengths, compensate for each of our weaknesses, and build on what works best for us. These guidelines remain my light and inspiration in setting up DAD training and expectations for my own role in this endeavor.

Admittedly, my brainstormed list of wishes and needs bring up all kinds of what-ifs. I worry about who will assist me or retrieve glucose tablets if no one is around besides Abbey. If I've "merely" done what most DAD trainers do—that is, teach my dog to give me a signal that my blood sugar is dropping, and that is all she does—how much help is that to me? What kind of trouble might unfold if there is no further intervention?

This sets my imagination into overdrive: a ridiculous scene unfolds—one I'd prefer not visiting as my precious dog taps my leg to alert me that my sugar is crashing and I am limp on the ground in the middle of my grocery store's parking lot as glucose tablets roll away from my hand just out of reach. By the time a bystander calls for an ambulance, I'm nearly gone—my faithful dog still by my side, poking me nonstop with her nose. People begin to circle us and praise my girl for her incredible dedication to the task as my rumpled body lies motionless. I can't hear—but I can imagine—what else they're saying just beyond earshot. Something about me. Something like, "'Too bad she didn't train that dog to do…more.'"

I don't yet have a plan or answer for this frightening but imaginary scenario that alternately generates peals of laughter and tears. But like all good and necessary things in the rhythm of life, it will surely come.

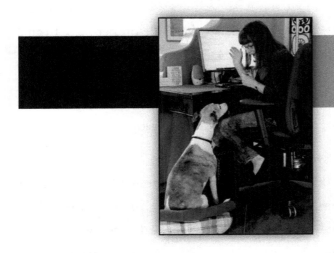

Chapter 6

I Am Not Alone

In the initial weeks spent trying to mold my youngest hound dog into an entry-level Diabetic Alert Dog, I believed many people probably laughed at the folly of my venture and may even have called me crazy; if not to my face, then certainly when my back was turned. I imagined them first saying, 'Who would be so silly as to choose a distractible hound as a service dog?' And secondly, 'What are the chances…?' I, myself, don't yet know the answer to this latter question.

In fleeting sweeps of paranoia, I second-guess simple facial expressions from my canine-working friends and mentors. None of my own efforts temper my questions, nor does my collective knowledge gained from working my dogs in agility, obedience, conformation and lure coursing. What rattles my own new resolve is the deep knowledge and experience held by other trainers. When my trusted agility instructor Hannah asks me how things are going in the "service dog training department," I rave about Abbey's newest skills. But catching a quick glimpse of a raised eyebrow belies the smile on her face. I can't help but wonder if she disbelieves me. This is someone who really knows dogs; she has trained and competed with them for years. This worry about her level of confidence in me sporadically upends my resolution when I allow it to carry more weight than it deserves.

This disconnect sweeps all reason, too, when I try to divine what Arie might really be thinking about Abbey's chances, when at the close of our lessons, my frazzled, nearly brain-dead dog rushes to the sliding glass door, barking mayhem death warnings to local flocks of mourning doves daring to intrude on her property and territory. At these times, I find myself desperately searching Arie's face for a clue as she stoically ignores Abbey's rowdy, most un-service dog-like behavior while writing up my next home-based training assignments.

Truly, I am too nervous to ask, yet too excited about Abbey's general progress, to openly share any of my own doubts about the logic of my goal. But then, to my surprise, just weeks into my training efforts, I find out I have company.

The e-mail from Arie comes out of the blue:

Hi Kat. Glad you got the book you ordered.

I have another client I'm starting to work with for DAD training (we're only about as far along as you and I are) for someone with Type 1 diabetes as well. They live near you, actually. I just wondered if you wanted me to give you each other's email address for support or anything . . . just a thought.

What in the world? It seems too strange a coincidence, but I'm not going to question fate. My heart soars. I send off a "quick okay" to Arie in my usual style.

> Yes, yes, yes! It would be great if you'd give them my name and email. I'll write something up and send it to you so you can forward it to them. THANKS!

Describing my response as open or exuberant or exhilarated is not an exaggeration. The fact is: I am all these things. But most of all, I feel hope to connect with someone nearby and on the same mission, which enhances the possibility to make a new and distinct set of friends.

"Bob," I shout. "You're not going to believe this! Come here and read this email." In my best teacher's voice, I add, "Now, please!"

He has no choice. Despite it being the end of a tiring workday, my level of excitement and insistent tone don't allow him to exercise his usual pattern of selective listening. To his credit, the man sometimes makes smart choices. He dutifully pads in his slippers to where I sit on the edge of my seat, at my laptop.

"Read this!" I repeat.

"Hmmm. Really?" he says. "That's interesting." A man of measured words. Why am I unsurprised at his cautious reaction?

"WHAT? Is that all you can say? Don't you realize how cool this is?" I demand.

As we talk—which really means that my enthusiasm about having a potential comrade holds my unfortunate spouse hostage—my mind races at the possibilities of connecting.

"You'll have to see what happens," he says in his usual astute manner.

It's true. I somehow manage to tap enough patience over the next few days to await Arie's response to my note. Everything in its own time, I remind myself. The delay seems interminable, but I do not want to push my luck.

At last, a reply finally appears on my phone. I peruse it in between teaching groups of students. Prospects of how and when we might meet and what we have in common tumble about in my head. Having these people as a touchstone in my journey helps me believe that I might begin to feel less isolated, just like the camaraderie of making friends at summer diabetes camp had helped me cope in the months and years after my diagnosis. Or like the startling discovery that my friend Rick, whom I met when we were twelve, had Type 1 diabetes just like me. This became a glue that bound us together for life. Just knowing he is in the world puts a smile on my face and makes a profound difference in how I face each day. Connections like these help me feel less alone; they allow me to approach a life marked by diabetes with just a little more determination and joy. It is no surprise that similar hopes stir at the cusp of Arie's introduction.

Sorry for the delay, but here are each other's email addresses so you can be in touch if you'd like. I'm sure you both have Facebook too that you can look each other up on.

☒ Kat (Kathy) with Abbey the whippet

☒ Ned (and his wife DeeDee) with Olive the black Lab

Also, Kat is planning to write a book about the journey of training a DAD, so you guys may also be in touch about that if you want.

> Thanks, and good luck. I'll be in touch with both of you again soon!

Yes! I couldn't wait to get home and send an email to DeeDee and Ned. But where to start? I ponder what information I'd be willing to share in our first interface. This is always the toughest question—how much is too much? Too personal? It's an issue that bears careful reflection. I jot another to-do on my daily list.

At home, my three dogs begin whining and pacing between where I am sitting at my desk and the kitchen, insisting on being walked. It's their nightly routine, but I brush their reminder aside and apologize, explaining that they have to wait. I see their shoulders slump ever so slightly as they move to lay down on their beds. Then I sit down with a cup of tea and tackle the email that will introduce two families—strangers—undertaking a common goal to surmount the same health issue. Or is it? All I've heard is that someone in this family lives with diabetes and that he or she needs a DAD. But what that really means, I don't know.

I face my next task; taking a chance to explain my own issues and reasons for wanting to train a DAD. That means wrestling with what I am willing to share in this initial connection. Finally, when the weak New Mexico winter sun surrenders its tease of flitting warmth as darkness pushes away the last remaining light of early spring, and the dogs have long given up their hopes for a walk by settling into soft cushions, my introduction seems ready.

> Hi DeeDee and Ned. You can only imagine how surprised I was to hear from Arie that another couple wants to train their dog to be a Diabetes Alert Dog! It surprised me even more that you may live nearby. My husband and I live in the area with our three whippets.

I don't know how successful I'll be in training my whippet Abbey, but I'm determined to try this and see how far we can get! My dog is 22 months old. I've taken her to obedience classes and work weekly on agility skills. My husband Bob and I have been living with whippets for many years, and Abbey is definitely a special girl, but it would be easier, I think, if we were to try training a Lab.

I am a long-time Type I and wear an insulin pump. I've been diabetic almost 50 years! That's unbelievable to me. For years, I was on multiple shots. Taking long-acting insulin was difficult, as it gave me very bad headaches and couldn't be adjusted to my varying day-to-day activities. So, I switched to a pump about 25 years ago, and I just started using a Continuous Glucose Monitor about 2 months ago.

Anyhow, can you tell me a little bit about you and how you decided to train your dog to help with diabetes blood sugar detection? Looking forward to hearing from you and sharing some of our dog-related DAD training stories!!!

There is no going back now. I do the only thing possible; I push forward, sensing there is so much more to understand beyond diligent training sessions and affirmation taken from Abbey's positive responses. Finding a touchstone in my intense pursuit promises to make working toward my DAD goal that much better. I know there are reasons beyond my immediate grasp that had set our two families on the same path—powerful ones that might inevitably link us. They merely lie in wait, tempting my imagination with delicious anticipation, and framed by the question singing in my heart: What if? This time, the question is filled with possibility. With nothing to lose, I suck in my breath, cross my fingers for good karma, and hit "send."

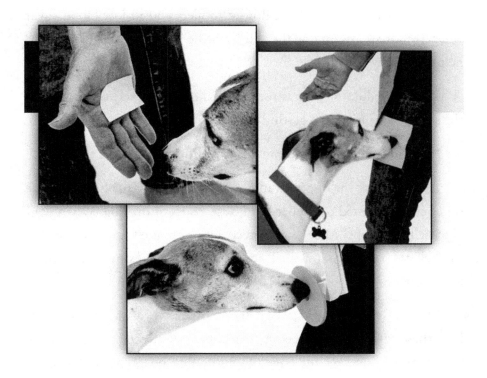

Chapter 7

Ding, Dong! May I Have Your Attention?

Despite my head holding so many questions about how to train my dog to connect alert signs to low blood sugar, this is pushed onto the back burner as I tackle my next task: finding a doggie doorbell. The device, which Arie had quickly demonstrated, is destined to be used by Abbey to tell me if my blood sugar crashes while sleeping or driving.

"Say what?" I retort to our trainer, emitting dubious, rapid eye blinks to emphasize my point. "Are you kidding?"

"No," Arie responds. "She'll need to alert you to low blood sugar when you drive. By ringing the bell from the back seat, she'll be able to help you know when to get food."

I am incredulous. This is something I'd never, ever, thought of in the scope of training and getting any potential help from my dog.

"But how?" Always the same question from this novice.

Arie smiles at the opportunity for an entrance. "Usually, the doggie doorbell is mounted on a board or box in reach of the dog. When your glucose level drops, Abbey will detect the scent. We'll train her to ring the bell at that time, and she'll touch it to let you know you need to treat for a low."

"Wow. Really?" I seem to be a master of few words at turning points like these; it feels like being somewhere between an inkling of understanding and on the edge of envisioning possibilities. These are mere sparks, really, but they begin to light up in the space between us.

I'd like to say I am delighted at the idea of my dog alerting me to low blood sugar in the car, but even trying to visualize it all, it is still a struggle to picture it in action. It's obvious that fully believing that this alert will pay off will demand more of my time and lots more training. I certainly have my doubts about a dog being able to link an alert signal to a doggie doorbell. That leaves me but one thing to do to counter my reservations: I plunge ahead to find out more about these contraptions, intending to order one and wait in a state of heightened skepticism until it is delivered into my hands, convincing me of its power.

But who knew such a plethora of options existed? At the click of the return button on my computer, a number of so-called 'best for pet' doorbells spring up in response to my search. There are so many: Bow

Wow Button, Pet-2-Ring, PoochieBells, and Pebble Smart, to name a few. The difficulty lies in which model to choose as I nervously read and reread detailed descriptions for each one.

Our trainer Arie had demonstrated the Pet-2-Ring, a perfectly workable model, its parts encased in a hardy, plastic rectangular box. It takes just a firm push of the paw on its lidded cover to make the bell ring. My hesitation in ordering one is its size—a bit long for easy mounting and access in the car—at least for how I envision my dog using it. I am not convinced she'll be able to push with enough force to make it work in a moving vehicle one hundred percent of the time.

After two weeks of research, a mountain of questions emailed to doggie doorbell vendors, and overzealous amounts of worry expended on the best model for Abbey, my decision comes down to two small points. One, a recommendation on purchasing the Pebble Smart Doggie Doorbell arrives from my neighbors and new DAD cohorts-in-training DeeDee and Ned. They love this device and tell me that their DAD-in-training has been successful at learning to push it with a tap of her nose. And two, there is the not-so-small fact that Pebble Smart's designer named it for his prized whippet Pebble. Let's face it; if you love your breed—as most of us do—there are no limits where such loyalties are concerned. You'll do anything to represent the dog breed you adore, and I certainly follow suit. It doesn't hurt, either, that the company's head graciously answers every question I email his way, letting me know that others successfully use his system, along with a multitude of different alert devices, for training various medical alert dogs.

Feeling increasingly comfortable about what might work for alert training with a doggie doorbell, this removes most doubts about my course of action. I happily order the Pebble Smart model from Amazon and wait with delicious expectancy.

The box arrives a mere four days later. Sitting at my front door upon my return from work, I dive into it. It seems simple enough: an electronic receiver bell fronted by a sunny, yellow disk attached to the transmitter box. A beautiful whippet, stamped on the box covers, greets me.

"Hello, Pebble!" I quip. "Thank you for coming to help Abbey learn how to ring a bell for a very good cause!"

Bob and I scan the instructions before inserting the required 9-volt battery. Once that is done, I rehearse the steps alone, hoping this dress rehearsal will keep me from confusing my dog. Finally, I pull a handful of small treats from the goodie jar on my kitchen counter—knowing all too well their persuasive power—before calling Abbey to me. And then I cajole, "Abbey, come!"

She slides toward me at full speed as if stealing a Little League base, nearly knocking me down; typical everyday enthusiasm from this red-brindled alpha girl. I recover, trying to follow the instructions to a "T" by holding onto the front of the transmitter box while my dog sniffs it. She gently brushes the disk, but no sound issues forth. Darn it.

I drop a small treat behind the yellow disk—something recommended in the directions. Let's go, girl. You can do this.

Abbey's nose pushes hard at the yellow disk, no doubt to reach the treat she smells but can't reach, behind it. Ding, dong. Ding, dong! Loud and clear.

"YES!" I tell her, using my voice as a marker. "Good girl!" These words take the place of a clicker used in Clicker training, and my positive tone works wonders. I then hand Abbey a treat since she can't get to the one tucked behind the yellow disk.

I am pleased to see she clearly knows that touching the doggie doorbell disk is like touching a contact lid on the agility field; something we'd already done many times. Such simple actions, when trained correctly, but so thoroughly understood and recalled by dogs. Just brilliant! The simple efficiency of canine intelligence never fails to delight me.

As Abbey discovers how to ring the doggie doorbell, connect my "yeses" to the desired behavior and then have her actions rewarded with treats, you can be certain that our sessions soon turn into a frenetic circus. The other two dogs in the house are not about to stand around waiting an imagined millennium for those hoped-for treats; they want in, too, and their drooling is prime physical evidence of their readiness to learn! That is how, despite Arie's reminder that only one dog in a household can truly fill the role of a service dog, I momentarily surrender and think, why not? I fervently hope the decision doesn't come back to haunt me.

Within minutes of Abbey pressing her nose to the yellow disk on the front of the small transmitter, her sisters Tess and Zoe join the frenzied search to be rewarded with treats too. The discovery process takes all of a few minutes—impressing even me. Soon my three dogs are vying for alpha status in their new nose-touching quest. This is a bit much to handle, so I call for reinforcement.

"Bob!" I exclaim in rising pitch, "Would you puh-lease come hold these crazy dogs?"

He strolls into the kitchen from the garage.

"Watch," I say, thrilled to have a helping hand in the midst of the drool- and fur-fest. "You won't believe how quickly they learned to do this."

One at a time, with the others pressing insistently forward, Abbey and Tess and Zoe put their noses to the yellow disk, sniffing for potential lurking treats, earning positive verbal markers for making the bell ring. Yours truly follows up each 'ding, dong!' with treats. The dogs are dizzy with excitement at this new game. Whippet tails swish about in delight. Three sets of eyes follow my every movement. Who wouldn't want to reach for success when playing a game and being rewarded with a yummy treat or catching a tossed toy every time you scored?

I smile in amazement at the simplicity of this initial training task while realizing how much work still lies ahead in joining Abbey's behavior to the real purpose for ringing the bell. I think, too, about Martinez and Barns' training recommendation: the 80% Rule, where any specific behavior being trained needs to be successfully demonstrated at least 80% of the time before moving on. It makes a lot of sense to build this kind of strong foundation based on consistent behaviors, and it definitely looks like we are on our way.

The next lesson with Arie—our fifth—goes well. Abbey demonstrates all the public access behaviors we've been learning. Our list includes commands like:

- Stay in your place. As in, lie down and stay on your rug near my feet or chair despite any ever-so-tempting distractions calling you elsewhere.

- Down. Meaning lie all the way down (no half-hearted, cheating "whippet downs" allowed) and stay there, near me, until released.

- Leave it. Don't bother with dropped or found food, children calling you to them, other people or any objects daring to pique your curiosity. And especially not your canine sisters who deserve their share of treats, too.

- Wait. An essential command to keep my dog patiently near me, giving me her full attention, letting customers walking in or out of a store unbothered, and as a precaution before moving around corners in order to keep both dog and handler safe.

- By my side. A helpful command meant to help maintain my dog's proximity to me without wandering or pulling away in all kinds of busy locations. Additionally useful for avoiding the temptation of packaged foods.

I'd learned all these commands are fundamental public behaviors for all service dogs, so it is a good place to begin working with mine. Arie would soon check for Abbey's grasp of these commands and more on our next session out in the real world. To pass, my canine companion needs to earn an 'always' or 'most of the Time' in fourteen categories and a whopping thirty-seven detailed behaviors found on the Assistance Dog Public Access Certification Test. Despite Abbey's solid background knowledge, we have our work cut out for us.

Helping Abbey understand Diabetic Alert Dog behaviors requires even more preparation than the group of public protocols in order to build her understanding of not only what to do, but when certain alert behaviors are necessary. Included in her DAD-training sessions, we practice a paw alert—"give me five"—keeping it in our repertoire for potential future training of that all-important high blood sugar alert. I reinforce the "touch" command every day, asking Abbey for a firm push into my hand with the snout. "Knee" or "nudge" requires a nose tap to the leg or knee area, with this behavior being drilled weekly—or more often.

While it may sound like a lot of pressure to maintain training, it's not; the sessions are conducted quickly and there are always oodles of laughter along with a deep sense of connection. I chose these alerts to be discreet but recognizable alert behaviors to signify dropping blood sugar. Abbey loves doing them, and to make it even more fun, I fashion games out of the commands and insert them into daily routines at unexpected times specifically to challenge her thinking. Boredom with too much routine is the direct opposite of what we strive to do, so I delight in mixing up the commands and tasks for her.

Still remaining in moving ahead with DAD training—collecting those all-important saliva samples. When my blood sugar plummets, this simple task is woefully complicated in the midst of symptomatic shaking and heart pounding. There is no doubt that "brain fuzziness," though temporary, remains an obstacle in the "saliva collection department" and is the primary reason for my lack of current samples. I resolve to outsmart the fugue of desperation that overtakes body and soul when my glucose level crashes by willing myself not to react in my usual pattern of rushing to pop candy or food into my mouth. THINK, I remind myself over and over again, or you'll never be able to start scent training Abbey.

As we walk out to Arie's car at the lesson's end, she notes how well Abbey and I are doing as a team. Encouraged, I divulge the question that has brewed in me for months.

"I'm happy with everything Abbey and I have learned," I begin, "but do you think I'm crazy trying to train Abbey to be a DAD?" Behind my question, a fervent hope: that Arie recognizes my girl's work ethic and abilities, similarly demonstrated by many breeds and mixed-breeds outside the Labradors and Golden Retrievers typically tapped in the service dog world.

Arie stares at me. Her direct gaze leaves nowhere to hide.

"No, I don't. I would have already had to tell you if I thought you wouldn't make it."

My heart jumps. I nod, realizing the weight of all my hopes channeled into this exceptional dog who feeds my spirit with her everyday antics and intense love. Something opens in me. Something deeper.

I can breathe now. Team Abbey has the gift of time—whatever is needed—to abandon ourselves to learning and practicing new skills on the service dog learning curve. As I begin to relax, my resolve shifts a bit and recognizes how vital it is to enjoy the journey, have more fun along the way and celebrate every step we tackle. I feel like a young child spinning round and round, arms outstretched, in dizzying, giggling circles of delight. I know, too, that I owe so much to my furry friend. She's given me the drive to take charge, to laugh, and problem solve, and to step into owning my path. All along, I've found myself drawing strength from Abbey's indomitable nature, and that's been good for me. At last, I have no doubts. I believe fully in our mission and each of us.

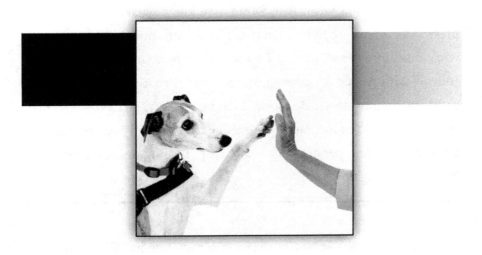

Chapter 8

Virtual Outreach

It doesn't take long to get an email response from my new DAD-cohort DeeDee and Ned. Sitting at my laptop to read their reply, adrenaline surges through my body in an overly-excited response, and I suddenly feel like a black-chinned hummingbird giddy on the first juices of native penstemons now rising in annual rebirth from my xeric gardens. There's no doubt where to place blame for the potential jump in blood sugar which will be inevitably triggered by the adrenaline pumping through my system. I lecture myself through flitting breaths: Calm down, relax and just read what they have to say. For me, the importance of being in the moment, while also keeping in mind the uber-importance of lowering stress levels, seem to require constant reminders.

Like now, with Abbey demanding cuddling and trying to push her thirty-two pounds onto my lap because my attention is momentarily diverted from the Queen Bee. Some may know what is meant by this nickname; others are free to guess. Sighing with impatience to find out what this family is all about, I force myself to shift my attention and snuggle with Abbey for a few minutes—not such a difficult task under ordinary circumstances. But soon, I tell her, "Sorry, girl. Now you need to let me be." She gives me a mournful gaze as I gently release her back onto the floor and pet her silky head before turning my attention to the awaiting message.

> Hi Kat.
>
> This is DeeDee. It is wild that you are so close by! We are on Janet Place just south of Lomas.

What? Just a neighborhood or so away! I call out to Bob to tell him about this circumstance—two families in such close proximity doing the same training with the identical trainer. Sometimes truth is stranger than fiction, and the coincidence makes me grin.

The email continues:

> My husband, Ned, was recently diagnosed with Type 1 about 2 years ago. We have learned a lot about diabetes very quickly. Ned uses long-acting insulin, but as you mentioned, he sometimes finds it does not adjust well to the variety of life. He tried regular insulin, but it caused him to crash, so he avoids taking it when he can.
>
> Ahh. I mull over this bit of news. Newly diagnosed with diabetes, Ned's pancreas might still be producing some insulin in order for him to have so many lows.

I understand the dread that accompanies these sudden crashes. Not fun. Scary, even. I've had many of these episodes marked by sweating, heart pounding and desperate panic. "Many" might amount to quite an understatement, as in fifty years of living with Type 1, I've averaged 1-3 major lows every week of my life with diabetes. That comes out to a preposterous number of incidents: an average of 2,600 on the low side to a high-end guesstimate of 8,000. Only seven times have I sought care in an ER with each of these incidents attributed to malfunctioning insulin pump equipment that triggered high glucose levels leading to ketoacidosis. The enormity of these numbers astounds me, proving how resourceful and strong the human body is—even in the face of major health challenges.

I want to email DeeDee a list of questions about the initial DAD training behaviors she chose, but I continue scouring the screen for more clues to better understand why her husband might need a service dog. Then, I see it; the answer is right in front of me. It's not much of a leap to understand the main issue that challenges him.

> Ned has very regular lows. We have had times where we discovered that he is at 62 while driving on the highway with the whole family in the car. He has gone as low as 35 but usually does not go below 60 or so. He drops to around 60 very regularly. We hope that if we can train Olive to alert, then he can prevent many of the lows.

I don't doubt the impact of Ned's struggle in trying to cope with the ups and downs of the disease.

Abbey pushes her way onto my lap again, but I stop her from jumping up this time, blocking out her insistent whining, exchanging the demand for my attention with a chew bone. I hope she'll ignore the fact that this isn't a completely fair exchange, but it is a necessary part of the current bargain since my priority is centered on the revelations spinning from my monitor. The exchange of a bone for a few moments of quiet is a quick fix, but with Abbey happily ensconced on her dog bed across from me, I hunker down to read more.

As to how we learned about diabetic alert dogs-

When we got Olive, my Lab, I was staying home and I trained as a therapy dog. We also did several obedience classes. I volunteered extensively at the animal shelter, so I have a lot of experience working with dogs.

When Ned had his health issues I went back to work and was not able to follow through on all the therapy training we did with Olive.

Hmm, not so different from me. I wonder how much of a common concern this is to everyone who lives with Type 1. Who wouldn't want an alert dog to help them avoid the unthinkable—whether it is ending up in the ER for treatment or never waking up at all from an extremely low glucose episode?

I reflect on all the training involved in my endeavor, wondering if this family might share some helpful insights for my own training venture. How, for example, did they start working with their own dog?

DeeDee addresses my questions one after another, her answers encouraging my chosen path.

We began trying to train Olive ourselves from what we had learned on the net. We had some success but we also really confused her.

I bought some books on training dogs for diabetic alert work and through sheer luck found Arie on the Internet. So far, the training has been going really well! We are ready to start with scent but cannot for a few months because (as often happens in life) we have too many things going on at once.

We aren't so far apart on the service dog training spectrum after all. DeeDee and I are both in the process of discovering, in spite of our research on how to train a DAD, that there is simply no substitute for hands-on training. Time and diligence are required. Consistent practice that builds on every skill, no matter how small, leads to success—or so it seems. We both realize that there are no shortcuts on the path to creating a working Diabetic Alert Dog.

I laugh at DeeDee's description of her family's busy lives, because it fully captures my own; working, raising a family and taking time to do interesting things that have shaped my journey. For me, and others living with any health issue, seamlessly integrating all these daily demands into everyday life is important. That is my numero uno objective. I just didn't realize, until now, that setting this goal would grow to include turning a regular pet into a "Superdog," of sorts.

DeeDee's email closes with a few details of their lives aside from Ned's journey with Type 1.

> We have two kiddos. Our daughter is 11 and our son just turned 9. We are so busy: boy scouts, girl scouts, gymnastics, skiing, camping, rock climbing with the family. I am hoping that having an alert dog will help Ned keep track of his blood sugar even when life is nonstop!
>
> I look forward to hearing how your training is going with your puppy.
>
> DeeDee

I hit "reply" and, ever so briefly, consider what to say. One question reverberates over and over in my head, so I ask DeeDee the single thought driving me forward with anticipation, trumping all others: When can we possibly meet?

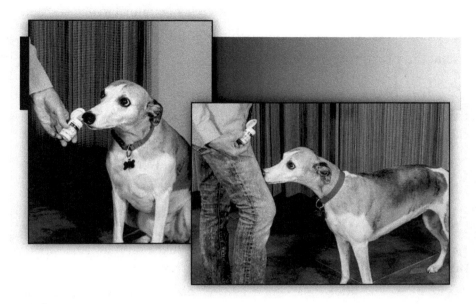

Chapter 9

Can You Smell Me, Pepé Le Pew?

Scent collecting looms large in my mind, making me wonder why I have put it off for so long. Of course, there are the supplies to marshal. I try rallying myself about shopping: what girl doesn't love to break away from everyday routine and search for treasures, even if they're for items as unglamorous as saliva sample repositories?

I'll admit, as the time arrives for collecting the scent samples that will allow me to train Abbey to recognize low blood sugar levels, my anticipation looms. So do old anxieties based on my very first fears about the feasibility of shaping my whippet into an effective DAD. My competitive determination to be successful is distracting me from digging in and breaking down the training into manageable pieces. The cynical, glass-half-empty part of my brain simply won't let me imagine how a sighthound can be thoroughly and reliably trained to detect scent. I remind myself that this line of thinking just might be a protective stance in case I happen to fail at my quest.

Time keeps on slippin', slippin', slippin', into the future. I wryly recall these ancient lyrics cemented without permission in my brain and see them for what they are; a motivator. A return to reviewing information in Martinez and Barns' training manual quickly fosters my flagging resolve.

I dive into the supply recommendations. The authors suggest picking up a number of items for scent training: unscented cotton pads; clean, small plastic tubes; and one or two tight-sealing freezer containers, like lidded glass food leftover dishes or heavy-duty plastic food storage ware, to contain and protect the scent samples. It's a simple list of materials, all easy to obtain. Once these items are gathered, I can begin collecting samples. At the ready on the home front, I also have a permanent marker for labeling the tubes and an accessible freezer in which to place the wrapped glucose scent samples. In my case, there are fewer items than others might need since I plan on collecting samples of only low glucose (versus low and high) levels. My "scenthound list" in hand, and my excuses neutralized, off I go to buy what is needed.

Over a week's time, I try to "catch myself" when my blood sugar drops. An insane task, apparently, and pretty much a dubious goal. Because every time my glucose falls, I have absolutely no supplies on hand. My difficulty in trying to not reach for food, as part of my typical emergency routine, just adds to the challenge. Most of my 'reactions' find my glucose dropping so rapidly that I can imagine eating the actual cotton swab intended to swipe my mouth for low blood sugar scent, if only it had even a hint of sugar on it, just on the hope that it might restore me and my crashing blood sugar to a state of normalcy. Remaining patient and calm, even when a sense of urgency for self-survival kicks in during lows, is going to be considerably thornier than ever imagined.

My gawky attempts to procure my first low blood sugar samples typically play out in a scene just like this one, where I'm driving home from work after a long day of teaching:

My CGM blurts out two long, slow beeps.

Oh no, why are you still beeping at me? Are those two long, slow beeps still telling me I have high blood sugar? Might be high blood sugar. Not sure.

Okay. Must check my sugar on my meter. Let's pull the car off the road. Oops; creeping above 195. Definitely outside my target zone. Oh brother; need extra insulin bolus. Now.

Pull back onto road.

Might as well run another errand. Can't eat dinner yet, anyway. Must wait for sugar to drop.

Back in the car, heading toward home.

More alerts from my CGM? Uh oh—three quick buzzes? That means I'm falling. FAST. Better watch out.

Nearing home. Hands shaking.

Must be low.

Need food.

NOW.

Anything will help.

Fumble around glove compartment.

Nothing.

I'm in real trouble. Ah, good. Here's something. Two old mints.

Rip wrapper. Shove into mouth. Ignore tacky plastic still glued to edges.

Phew. That should hold me.

Wait a minute! I ate before getting out of the car and swabbing my mouth for low blood sugar scent?

What an ignoramus.

Sitting outside my driveway with my glucose level now rising, the luxury of clear thinking is restored once again, and I realize my attempt to gather a sample has been thwarted. How am I to remember to swab my mouth before eating something when I'm shaking so hard, I can't think beyond the moment, and my scent collection supplies—neatly lined up on a counter inside my home—are nowhere within reach?

This scent trapping business most definitely requires another plan. My next strategic move is to capture a low on the home front. An easier task since supplies are nearby, but I'll still have to contend with some plummeting lows driving me to grab any source of simple carbohydrates before my conscious brain can wrestle with letting go of its "IMMINENT DISASTER: EAT NOW!" cry.

My first home-capture attempt, and most subsequent tries, unfold like this episode as I prepare to launch myself into the garden:

Okay, let's test your glucose level. 157? Perfect for a few hours of digging and bed cleanup. In fact, have a small cookie, if you want one.

Sunscreen? Check.

Hat for shade? Don't want one.

Food or sugar? Nope, I'm home. Can just walk inside when I need something. Whew, I feel great! Two garden beds filled in with annuals for spots of needed color. Now to fertilize the veggies and roses.

Hmmm. Starting to slooow down.

Dang it. Numb around mouth and lips.

Aww, don't be a weakling. What are you worried about? There's more to do. Keep going. You have more in you than this!

Okay. I'll keep going. I'm no quitter.

Where's that hose? Have to water down everything. Then I can stop and get something to eat.

Sounds like a plan.

Uh oh. Vision closing in on me now.

Go inside.

Help.

I say it out loud to no one. The supplies are inside on the counter, and my brain wrestles between pushing me to shove food into my mouth before I imminently fall over, or taking a chance and allowing me to think through collecting a scent sample. Somehow, today, I move against the grain of my standard emergency-response repertoire to grasp food, and I sit down.

You can do this, my conscious brain—the weaker one by now—coaches. Then, you can eat.

Open blood sugar meter. Grab lancet. Wipe dirt off finger. Push. Again. Ouch.

45? Oh boy. Can I eat now?

Uh uh. Not yet. Take that cotton swab. Rub it inside your cheeks. Over your tongue. Side one. Side two.

My mouth is dry and the cotton sticks to it in tufted pieces.

Oh no, not cotton all over my tongue! I hate that.

So what? Don't be a ninny. Spit.

Now? Can I eat now?

Almost.

Put that cotton pad into the empty glucose strip container. Pick up the permanent marker. Write blood sugar. The date.

Are you kidding me? I'll never make it.

C'mon, you drama queen. You are almost done and ready to go.

Eye roll. Disbelief at this one-sided conversation.

Push, push, push. C'mon and finish this task for the first time.

I write—weakly. '45.' Then, below it: 5/29.

The recesses of my brain scream.

Wrap it. Freeze it.

No. It will wait. Candy. Juice.

My narrowing vision wins out, and I grab for the nearest fix as I allow myself quick kudos.

YESSS! You finally did it!

I take a well-deserved slump onto a nearby chair to shovel food in. So good. So grateful. I wait for the shaking to subside.

That's how the first low glucose sample, to be used for DAD training, made history—at least in my household. Not quite as difficult as I'd imagined but definitely a challenge between warring parts of the brain and my normal routines. This initial success instills elation, and it provides me with a model for capturing the future samples in my DAD training kit.

Once several vials are collected and on hand, training sessions begin. Abbey and I work together dozens of times each week at alerting to low blood sugar samples. Honestly, she seems a bit bored with it all, and it is no wonder. I discover that this amount of introductory training isn't necessary. As Martinez and Barns note, the magic of imprinting scent happens within three sessions. Trying to earn points for being an overachiever, as in my case, is a waste of energy toward helping my crafty canine learn and master helpful DAD behaviors.

I have chosen a hand touch as Abbey's initial alert, followed by a knee poke. We practice these until my happy dog performs the touches regularly. Treats, along with changes to my requests, like playfully turning my stance 180° from her approach, keep her engaged.

"Abbey, touch!" I sing. And sure enough, she jabs her damp, pointy, sweet whippet nose into my right palm.

"Knee, Abbey, knee!" I urge. Her nose brushes my right thigh just above my knee. I work several times a day to get her to touch me more firmly and with some chutzpah. A weak alert can be too easily misinterpreted. When this command is fully understood, I introduce a slight change, hoping Abbey won't flinch at the modification.

"Nudge, Abbey," I tell her. She looks up at me for a moment. All it takes to reassure her and smooth the transition to the command alert word recommended by Martinez and Barns is tapping on my leg a few times.

"Yes, Abbey," I repeat, my excited voice stretching a near half-octave above normal range. "Nudge." And that does it! If only every part of training a dog could be this easy.

Not long after this success, a problem appears: Abbey seems even more disinterested. To counteract her marked disdain for alerting to my nonstop shoving of frozen scent samples practically up her nostrils, I take a new tact. I begin to turn the detection of low glucose into a game by hiding the containers in pockets, waistbands, on table tops and even under the sofa. This works, more often than not, evidenced by Abbey's stronger nudges. I can't help but be grateful for those blessed canine olfactory sensors—so superior to a human's!

Abbey continues to learn. Based on this record, my hopes remain high.

I awake one morning with Abbey curled beside me. Asymptomatic for any glucose abnormalities, I reach for my bedside home test kit and load a hefty bead of finger blood onto the awaiting strip.

"What the hey?" I say to no one in particular.

A reading of forty-three miffs me. I feel like I've been backhanded by an opposing team sneaking up on me. And then, I sit bolt upright, realizing Abbey is beside me and nothing is happening—at least from her! Me? My brain is still, somehow, functioning sufficiently—and I am not at all pleased. I lower myself onto the bedcovers like a slithering snake, grabbing her face and pulling her toward me to smell my wrist and mouth.

"Lazybones," I growl, "not doing your job today? Off duty? You must be dreaming about chasing wild bunnies or roadrunners. What are you thinking?"

She doesn't stir or give any alert whatsoever. No touch into my hand. No nudge at my leg. Just a deep moan of happiness as she resettles alongside me in bed and nestles her long nose into most of my soft, down-filled pillow.

"Bob," I call out to the sound of water hitting glass. He is in the shower, so I make my way to the bathroom and mutter a few epithets about time wasted on dogs who would rather sleep and not do their jobs. Along the way, I dryly wonder if this could be anyone's scenario from which the phrase "Let sleeping dogs lie" possibly came, even though I know better. This morning, though, it is unequivocally mine.

"Hey," I say as my husband exits the shower, "do you think I'm wasting my time? That stupid dog didn't even sniff me this morning." I nod toward the ignorant beast in question. "What good is she to me, anyway?"

"Calm down," he replies. "Blood sugar low?"

I nod while Abbey rolls over on her back, legs pumping in the air as she happily dream-chases some moving life form in the eat-or-be-eaten kingdom. There is no question she is intently enjoying her time somewhere—just not here with me.

"I'll get you something. Hold on."

He walks toward the kitchen, towel wrapped around his torso and dripping feet leaving outlines on the floor. A minute later, as my mouth opens like a baby chick's, he pops a large piece of cookie right in.

"Mmmm," I mumble. "Yum." I am not so far gone that a delectable treat can't stir me.

"More practice, I guess," he notes.

"Yep," I agree. "But how are we going to get her to do this?" The dream of my own DAD being trained to bring me the suddenly acceptable couple of small cookies to treat my "lows" has an undeniably strong appeal at moments like these, even if it's a mere mirage.

But is it truly just a fantasy? I can't help smiling and wishing for more help in treating dangerously low blood sugars. Any person bringing me something yummy to treat crashing sugars has always engendered a deep sense of gratitude, and many points, in the game of life. I find myself obsessively tackling how I might train my DAD to meet this very real necessity head-on. If she could be trained to help me by fetching glucose tablets, it would be akin to something like divine intervention; a true miracle. I make a mental note to reward Abbey, that is, once she begins to tap into the brain cells that promise she'll keep her end of our bargain. I sense that accruing points matters, even to dogs, who always seem to know when you owe them. Maybe my wish will come to fruition sometime down the road, but for now, it's back to boot camp for me and my precious little beastie.

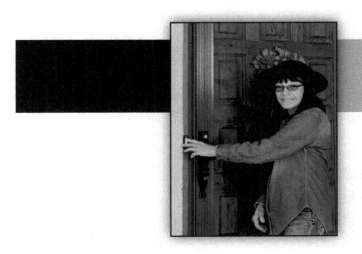

Chapter 10

Another Dad Household

If anyone noticed that life moves at a crazy pace in my own uber-Type A schedule-driven home, they'd be off by a light year compared to the forces radiating from DeeDee and Ned's household the Saturday afternoon we stop in to meet them and their puppies. Buzzed and besieged with energy and activity? These words barely describe the experience my husband and I encounter upon meeting the family I have longed, for weeks, to visit.

"Bob," I say, "What would you think about walking a neighborhood or two over to their place?" It's a Sunday, but work on our home improvements never seems to be done. Even on a sweet spring day like this—filled with classic, bright, billowing clouds under the sparkling sapphire sky that New Mexico is known for. Those siren skies beckon me to stop for ice cream on the swing or take a hike with the dogs. Or head out for a walk to meet this new DAD-focused family.

We are up to our elbows laying tile and mortaring an outside kiva fireplace and patio wall. Although I insist in the heat of the afternoon to make time for a visit, Bob has other thoughts.

"We need every minute we can get," Bob replies. "How about if we quit working and clean up at 2:30? Then we'll drive over."

"All right," I answer, glad he agrees to go at all. Between DeeDee and Ned's schedules with their kids, and ours, it has been nearly impossible to find a date that works.

We finally tuck our pack into the outdoor kennel, despite their protests, and drive to our destination. I ring the bell.

DeeDee greets us.

"Well, finally." She smiles. "Hello."

She explains that her family has just returned from a birthday party, and they are preparing to host an evening gathering for friends in a few hours.

"Come in, come on in," she says in a rush. She sweeps her arm toward the kitchen.

"Lots of people coming and going today, but come on out back. Ned's there with a friend."

"Great," I reply.

DeeDee says, "We were in the middle of training Olive when we decided we just needed to have a litter of puppies. Once these pups are weaned, plans are to resume Olive's DAD training."

I nod, aware that most dogs training as service dogs are spayed or neutered to remove many distracting factors from their new lives where they must be focused 24/7 on readily assisting their handlers. Tucking my questions aside, I say nothing, quietly noting that it is impolite to probe into their reasons for breeding their intended DAD.

Unable to resist the lure of puppies, though, and with not a peep to clue us in as to where they might be located, I ask, "Where are they?" Weren't eleven pups bound to be in sight, crawling everywhere and anywhere?

"Back this way. Follow me," she answers as she moves to the back door.

We trail DeeDee through the front den and kitchen, out into the backyard, and toward the garage. It's obvious this space offers not only quiet but shelter from the glaring afternoon sun.

While I want to see the pups, my main reason for visiting is the chance to chat and make connections. At the top of my list is my hope to talk privately with Ned about his experiences living with Type 1.

But I defer and answer, "That sounds great," in as nonchalant a cover-up as I can muster. Bob and I try to keep up and follow DeeDee's hurrying form. Ned—whichever one he is of the two tall men standing in the backyard—is engaged in deep conversation. DeeDee ushers us past them toward the garage without stopping to interrupt or make introductions. We walk along a pathway formed by pavers where shade offers welcome shelter from May's warming mid-afternoon temperature. In that shadowed overhang, solid black puppies are plopped like randomly lobbed inkblots from a paint splatter wheel. My heart jumps at the sight, and I kneel gently near one of the scattered litter.

It is then that the doorbell rings.

"Oops," says DeeDee. She cranes her neck back toward the house.

"Must be my sister. Sorry. We didn't expect so many people to come at the same time. Go ahead. Pick up the pups. I'll be back in a few minutes."

She shrugs her shoulders and zips in the direction from which we'd just come—toward the kitchen, leaving us alone.

And there they are, strewn in front of us, forming a distinct, albeit irregular, path of black markings all the way into the garage. After the strenuous competition of nursing, they'd tumbled, obviously depleted, into a well of sleep. Not one stirs at our encroaching presence. Their weary mother, the partially-trained Diabetic Alert Dog, lies in the choicest spot; on a bed of cool pine chips spread onto the floor of her whelping box. She manages to open one bleary eye to check out the approaching strangers before slumping back to rest.

DeeDee reappears, bends down, and scoops up one pup, handing him to me as promised. This one feels as heavy as a stuffed sack of potatoes, albeit much softer to the touch, which is surprising for approaching just eight weeks. He breathes deeply and evenly, limp in my arms, as the potion of sleep holds him captive. I glance at Bob for a reaction that might cue me in to any crack in his earlier resolve to only "take a peek" at the pups, but I see nothing. No sign of weakening. No chance of "yes." I can always hope, but today, window shopping is my only option.

I reluctantly place the unresponsive pup on the soft pine chips at my feet. I wonder, looking at him, if he or his mother would awaken to give an alert if my blood sugar dropped? It seems rather unlikely.

"Sorry," says DeeDee. "Hopefully they'll be up in a bit and you'll be able to see their personalities."

"So," I venture, "have you been able to do any more training with Olive?"

"No. We want to get back to it, but our sessions with Arie have to wait until the puppies are gone," DeeDee answers.

I toss out another question as DeeDee sweeps back through the yard. "How far along are you with your DAD training?"

"We were making good progress. She was alerting to samples Ned collected. Low and high blood sugar."

"Wow," I state. "That's impressive. Maybe you can give me some pointers."

"Well, one thing we did was to place scent samples next to the puppies almost from the time they were whelped," she adds.

"Really? What does that do?"

"All the puppies are now imprinted with scents for lows and highs. We haven't trained them with it, but they're used to the smell," DeeDee explains. "That's a good start, and it makes training easier."

"That's really cool," I reply.

These pups, I note, might just be that much smarter than the average canine. I wonder if they have any advantages over my own dog, being that they are acquainted with two different scents for high and low glucose levels.

My thoughts meander while yet another couple strides through the kitchen door to greet DeeDee in the yard. We are introduced by name, but neither Bob nor I have any clue as to their relation to the hosts. The mix of people stopping in, by this time, is growing exponentially. Identifying relationships to people so new to us is an enigma. In fact, I am still waiting to discover who Ned is in the mix of multiple visitors.

As DeeDee walks with us toward her friends and family, she asks, "Maybe you know of some people who would like a Diabetic Alert Dog and would be willing to do more training with them?"

"I'll check around. I can talk with the Director at our area's American Diabetes Association (ADA) office or someone connected to the local Juvenile Diabetes Research Foundation (JDRF) to see if they can put the word out. And I know several friends and families in the city who might be interested."

"It would be so nice if a few of these puppies could go to nearby homes," DeeDee says. "Would make it easier to stay in touch."

I nod in agreement.

"C'mon," she says, "let's go meet Ned."

Ned, it turns out, is the tall, thin man who now walks toward us and away from all the visitors. He mentions that he works for a design firm but says nothing about his diagnosis or training the dog. There are so many questions I want to ask, but this just isn't the right day.

As the doorbell rings yet again and another couple enters the house, I walk toward Ned and DeeDee's kids. Cydney, age 11, and Milo, nine, sit on the den sofa, deftly oblivious to the hubbub that surrounds them. They are focused in their own little bubble; a world in which Milo avidly plays a game on his iPad, and Cydney immerses herself in a book. When DeeDee introduces us, they scowl at the interruption. I give them a quick hello and step away.

With all the commotion, it feels like we've been dropped softly, ever so quietly, toward earth in a magical hot-air balloon ride, only to be interrupted by loud bursts of propane and hard skips along thirsty ground as we brace ourselves for a bumpy landing. The buzz of multiple conversations and distractions is palpable, and it grows increasingly apparent that my hopes for a deeper connection have to be put on hold. At least for now.

Bob and I leave the visit with our new cohorts less than an hour after our arrival. I am disheartened by the chasm between my initial goals of sharing some of our experiences on handling the obstacles of living day-to-day with diabetes and a few training tips for our dogs, versus the reality we had just encountered.

"What just happened here?" I ask as we climb back into the car.

"Life," he says.

I take a deep breath and recall all the forces competing for our attention when we, too, had children at home.

"Doing ok?" Bob asks. I nod and give him a wan smile.

Days later, a follow-up email arrives from DeeDee.

It was so great to meet you the other day. Sorry things were so crazy at the house when you came by.

If you are up for another crazy visit, this weekend we are starting to send puppies home so hopefully it will be the last weekend we will have most of them. If you are interested in playing with puppies and can come by some time, let us know.

:)

I reach deep inside myself thinking about the purpose of our visit and what we had been able to share. More clarity surfaces away from the whirlwind we experienced. What I settle on is this: meeting each other was a positive start, and because our families are still connected by a similar challenge and journey, there will be other opportunities where we can come together again. I look forward to those times.

Seeing that litter of black-as-ink puppies, with all their promise of intelligence, companionship and future glory, was nothing if not splendid. So much potential. In true form, I am touched by this precious, new life. My imagination is swept away, too, visualizing working with them, tumbling along on an agility course or in rally and obedience. I even dare to let my mind's eye sweep into the purposeful, satisfying work of shaping them into DADs and being a member of one of these human-canine teams. And for one crazy, feel-good moment, despite the imagined resistance my alpha Abbey-girl would surely voice, I find myself fervently wishing I could adopt them all.

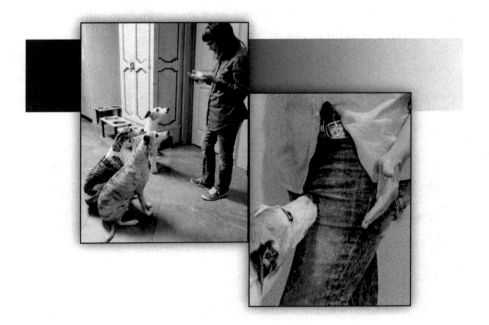

Chapter 11

A Day In The Life Of Dog & Handler

We are on the fast track now, and the right one, too. Our days begin to revolve around DAD and public access behavior tasks. Training specific behaviors ensues a minimum of twice each day. Squeezing in commands between my own writing sessions, when I take the dogs outside, even while preparing dinner. The quick pace keeps Abbey interested in learning, and me, on my toes.

A morning session might contain fifteen or more randomized commands that now include reviews for basic obedience, agility, public access and DAD training. It typically rolls out like this:

"Good morning, Gabby-Abbey, Tesla Tsunami and Zoe Rose! Let's get breakfast. Ready?" All three dogs watch me, quivering and waiting for a physical or verbal signal. I move my hand away, signaling them to move forward, accompanying it with a verbal release.

"Okay, let's go!" We all pad to the kitchen, doggie tails wagging ever faster. They know their favorite treats are a "given" after training time.

"Abbey, Tess, Zoe: Come front! Good girls."

I lift my hand up and say, "Sit." Then, "Let's try this again—sit by my side." They comply.

"Okay now. Watch me." I look directly at each dog to make sure she is attentive.

"Are you ready?" I ask. "Okay, swing!"

These commands and a hand movement tell all three dogs to rotate counter-clockwise from an in-front sit position. They park their skinny whippet rears in a heel position by my left side.

Then, I give a verbal marker, praising them all but paying particular attention to Abbey's execution, knowing she'll be tested several times and must meet qualifying standards for service dogs.

I'm happy with the drill and sing out, "Good girl!" The phrase makes me laugh out loud at my own joke; all of my hounds believe I'm speaking directly to each of them. That makes me fall over laughing for the umpteenth time, particularly at the sight of my pack jockeying for position and treats at my side.

Giving up for the moment, I move toward the pantry and dip into the dog kibble. As I come back out, all three panting dogs wait there, tails wagging, tongues flapping and eyes fixated as if they haven't seen me for hours.

"What is it, girls?" I ask. "You want to do more?"

I need a mental break, but my devotees won't let me off the hook. We move back into the kitchen.

"All right, let's ring the doggie doorbell! Ready?"

Tails wag. I hold the doorbell against a cabinet at various heights.

"Ring the bell!" I say, but no prompt is really needed.

Two noses push the yellow disk. Ding, dong! Treats abound, praise swirls and more tidbits appear, tossed into the air, for them to catch. This sequence puts into practice our car alert, which I have yet to team with a low glucose scent. For now, it's enough that we're learning to ring the car alert marker.

"That's enough," I say. "Breakfast time now."

I fill their dishes with half-servings of kibble and a sprinkle of grated cheese.

"Wait," I command, watching like an on-the-edge competitive agility coach, making sure they don't break their stay. Satisfied, I issue, "Okay. Bingo. Eat." All three dogs dive into their bowls at the magic release. When they finish licking up their last morsels, they gape expectantly at me.

Really? You want more? But their high-level expectation is persuasive enough to make me reconsider my desire to sit at my laptop.

"Ready to go out? Let's find the turtles."

We head through the garage to the enclosed rescue-box turtle yard—all the safer a route to keep the dogs near me. They wait, peering inside, for me to unlatch the gate, hoping to be the first to detect any in the paddock. I swing the gate open, and Abbey rockets into the yard.

"Gentle!" I warn.

She barely glances at me and heads off, sniffing for turtles hidden under layers of leaves and dirt. I spot a few of the larger ones while the dogs search for those less obvious. Hami! Chelsea! I greet two of the largest females who are lobbing mealworms like heavy, monsoon-generated raindrops, and ripping apart greens pulled from the nearby garden.

The dogs are having a heyday digging and jumping into a closer bed brim with fragrant herbs. I fill water into galvanized bowls for the turtles, all the while keeping a keen eye on Abbey, who needs extra attention with the "Leave it!" command. She resists my direction, bounding further into the yard, delightedly tracking down Hunter, the smallest of the concealed reptiles. She can't resist flip-playing with him, demonstrated just once, but reason enough for me to step into her path to safeguard the year-old hatchling.

Abbey is also prone to stealing choice bits of food, such as mushrooms and ripe strawberries, from the turtles' feeding bowls. Mastering the "Leave it!" command is critical, as she will soon accompany me into busy stores and must learn to ignore people or plates of food with no undue attention (or drool). Practicing this command while visiting the reptiles is an excellent routine as long as I'm fully attentive to her antics.

Once the turtles are fed and checked, we move to the other side of the yard to practice agility. These are activities Abbey loves; agility allows for movement through various obstacles and encourages both speed and quick thinking. Here at home in but a narrow slice of yard, our pace is much slower than at a practice or trial, but it still allows for a change in routine.

"Down, Abbey," I say. "Wait for your turn."

These commands are not only agility and obedience commands, but public access (PA) behaviors, too. The diva isn't pleased; she wants to be first, always. Finally, after Tesla and Zoe have practiced their routines, she reaps her turn.

"Jump. Teeter. Go tunnel," I call out.

She obliges in beautiful leaps and dashes, basking fully in the spotlight of attention and foreseeable training treats.

When we finally reenter the house, I open the freezer and pull out a frozen vial marked with scent from one of my low blood sugars. It sits thawing on the counter for ten minutes while I glom onto my emails to get them out of the way.

Then I step back into the kitchen after distracting Abbey with a chew treat and place the vial into my palm so it's not easily visible to her. My goal is to have her register the scent—not the vial. I tuck it into my pants pocket and walk back to the computer, praying Abbey will come up to me and give me an alert—either a hand touch or a nudge on my leg or knee. She doesn't. I am disappointed but note that she is heartily chewing a dental toy—one which my husband had given her. I silently chastise him with a "bad boy!" and then gently coax it from my dog.

"Give, Abbey, give it to me. It's yours, I promise. Abbey can have it back later, okay? Give."

I stare her down until she begrudgingly drops the chewie into my hands. She's not happy, but at least she's watching me. I parade back and forth in front of her, hoping the scent from the hidden scent sample will somehow waft out and clue her in. Miraculously, it does! I don't know how, because despite the number of times I've tried to sense what she smells from my sample, I can't detect anything. She, however, takes a step toward me. And another.

A nudge. Then a touch.

"Good girl!" I say.

Her tail wags as she waits for her treat. Again, she nudges my leg.

Yes! Two treats earned for that work. I toss one and then another extra high into the air, making a game of it. She seems happy now, but I am ecstatic. I close up the vial, snap it into its two outer protective containers and back into the freezer for the next scent training session.

I move on to my morning tasks and give Abbey some respite from her learning. Truth is, she might be willing to perform these tasks all day if the routine is varied and infused with fun, but I'm the one who actually needs the break. I resolve to pick it up again this afternoon or tonight. To let her know she can trust me and that I haven't forgotten my promise, I hand over her gnawed chew bone.

"Good girl," I sing for the twentieth time today.

This is the way the morning's motivational training session takes place; one that combines obedience, agility, service dog and DAD commands. I mentally check off one successful coaching interaction of the two or three we do most days. Some days, there's no time at all. But it's all good, as long as we keep moving forward and consistently address behaviors meant to connect thinking with actions.

Pacing Abbey's lessons has taught me a great deal in the short but intense four months we've spent training. I find that every session with my girl, even those squeezed into my busiest days, have a few things in common that guide me and build a strong foundation for every step in DAD training. Consistency and patience, on my part, are crucial. Stressed or deprived of a good night's sleep? Far better to skip a training session than to push ahead. A go-to strategy that I've found works wonders is rehearsing steps in practice runs by envisioning each task mentally and carrying it out physically, all without my dog. It is also helpful to think about my breed's specific needs; how she learns best, what motivates her, and what things distract her. As I push myself to think like a whippet, it is often amusing, and usually a joy, to work on modifying tasks I'm teaching based on how Abbey thinks and reacts to stimuli and commands.

I am beginning to understand and accept that everything happens in its own time. Sometimes, good things—even great things—come from simple understandings. I know that these underpinnings are an important key to grasping the service dog world and the larger, everyday world within which Abbey and I interact. Our new skills as partners give strong wing to hope and success. From this flank, I am able to envision what can be accomplished as Team Abbey moves full steam ahead. The finish line will come but lingering long enough to lap up each step of this journey is proving to be mighty remarkable and juicy, too.

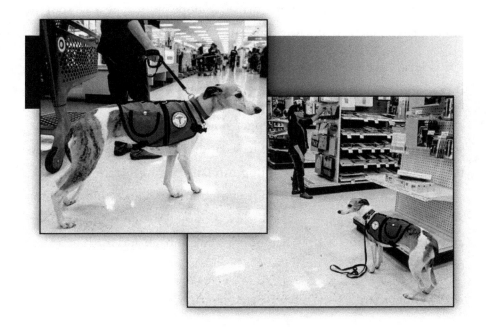

Chapter 12

Mom And DAD's Day Out

Each day spent training my sighthound, the seer of all things and whose job it apparently is to make sure that I, too, am aware of every change in routine she so keenly detects, brings both joy and challenges. But a new worry emerges as we prepare for entering the public arena in the first one of two formal practice runs with Arie. I reread the PA standards and visualize what we'll be asked to do. I think about the deep level of awareness needed for me to keep my dog safe when visiting public spaces. Mini-practice sessions abound as we prepare for our first big day under Arie's keen eye.

The first formal drill takes place one humid afternoon in June. I drive Abbey to a local Target and wait in the car as instructed by Arie.

Soon, my mentor's apple-red SmartCar bops into a nearby spot to announce her arrival. She waves us out.

"Heya," she greets me with a huge grin. "Let me show you a few things you need to know to get a service dog in and out of a vehicle."

She moves to the rear passenger door where my dog watches us, seemingly spellbound. For a split second, I wonder if Abbey looks pleased as she awaits two bumbling humans communicating our next steps that are all about her. I move to open the door while signaling Abbey to stay. One glance at her beloved trainer, the giver of all praises, and she gains steam, her tail beginning to whip back and forth in a state of near-ecstasy.

"Whoa, there," I warn her. "Steady, girl. Stay."

"Good," Arie comments. "We always want our dogs to exit the car quietly and in control, ready to obey. So, let's give her an idea of what we want by releasing her and putting her in a heel position."

I nod in understanding and open my mouth to do just that. As I inhale a few deep breaths of air to allow myself thinking time before issuing this seemingly simple command, Arie's question interrupts my planned move.

"First, have you checked the pavement to see how hot it is?"

"No," I reply, discombobulated at my lack of attention to such an important detail. "But good idea," I quickly say.

Kneeling down, I touch the asphalt with the back of my hand. While prostrate, I grab a silent chance to pray to any nearby spirits guarding dog lovers in the universe. *Please let me save face and not make too many handler errors.* I hope against hope that they somehow stick by me for guidance. Already, my temples are beginning to pulse at this first small detail I've forgotten.

"Doesn't seem too warm to me. Should I bring her out of the car now?"

Arie nods.

Mustering a clear voice, I give her release word.

"Okay, Abbey. Bingo."

She directly observes me, now at the ready. "Come. By my side, girl."

She jumps down, tail wagging in rapid circular beats, moving quickly into heel position. Pride surges through me; I can't help feeling it, and my sense of worry lifts. I breathe an audible sigh of relief as we move toward the large electronic glass entry doors and joyously bound inside, ready for the next challenge.

"Wait. Let's try that again."

The voice that slowly drifts into my consciousness and freezes me pretty much in mid-air and mid-step is Arie's. Gentle, but insistent. *Uh oh. What now?* I stop and glance back at my trainer, who is still outside the sliding entryway and at least four giant leap-frog steps behind.

"The right way to enter a store is to wait for exiting customers to move past you before you go inside." She shrugs in apology.

"Really?"

"Yep. It's a safety measure for the dog, and it gives you time to assess the situation with who's exiting the store, letting their carts get past you, that kind of thing."

"Phew," I say. "Okay, Abs, let's try this again."

We shift backwards in an attempted redo, much like reverse-shuffling a deck of cards. Abbey needs help recalling how to move in reverse, unlike her older sister Zoe Rose, a master of rally moves like this one.

"Back," I order, "back, back, back." I step directly into Abbey's chest and her path, crowding her so that she has no choice but to step backward.

A silver-haired man watches, quietly smiling his approval and bemusement, before passing us and waving as he exits the store. Once he moves on, we look right and left and then ahead, scouting potential obstacles. When all these tiny steps are mentally checked off, I take another deep breath and we finally step inside.

"Abbey, slow," I remind her. The Queen Bee needs a few hard tugs to cue her not to surge ahead in her typical, exuberant manner; to stay with me in her defined role.

We move, as instructed, up and down a few aisles, each time approaching a block of summer fun items. *Doing well.* I smile.

"Ehhhhh!" Arie honks, nasal-like, just like a game show buzzer. Caught through the perspective of my peripheral vision, she is smiling.

But I, for one, am definitely not. The sound reels me into the moment and out of my general happy-we're-doing-pretty-well status. It is then that I catch what prompted the negative sound; Abbey's long, pointed snout pushing insistently toward the display of a dozen or more "grab and go" snack packages, hung precisely at the improper level for a dog's sniffer to ignore. They're definitely exuding an open invitation to a dog like mine, in particular. *I only glanced away for a few seconds, and this is how she betrays me?* I have to chuckle as I yank her back with a "No, stay by my side." The true nature of canines, in time, consistently reveals its hand. If only I can learn to better anticipate the power of this phenomenon and apply it every time I enter the dog-training arena!

Tweaking my thinking makes a difference. We weave in and out of row upon row of clothing and other merchandise. Abbey stays on my left, leaving enough leeway to move with me, as we move through aisles. She carefully walks by my side, checking to see what I want her to do by seeking my lead and verbal commands.

She sits and waits on command and even drops down into a 'stay in your place' while I perform the charade of perusing merchandise. *Is it wrong that my heart swells with pride for one quick moment?*

At Arie's urging, I check my girl's startle reflex and recovery time by selecting and dropping three shelved items, each heavier than the last. The goal is to help Abbey accustom herself to unexpected sounds in busy, public places so she doesn't overly startle. Some level of reaction is normal and acceptable, but service dogs cannot exhibit edginess at sudden noises, nor should they be unable to return to performing the tasks they were trained to carry out. I start by selecting three flat items: an art kit, a notebook and a larger boxed set of file folders. I hold my breath, wait for Arie's signal, and drop them one by one. All good. This is an enormous obstacle, and it's thrilling to see that my dog doesn't exhibit avoidance behaviors—much unlike a few of my other more movement-prone, reactive whippets.

The next public access task Arie brings to my attention assesses my dog's ability to stay while I move some distance away from her in the store. Arie checks on any need for additional training on these wait-stays. Once again, I hold my breath while walking away from Abbey.

"Abbey, sit." I tell her. She ever-so-slowly, whippet-style, backs down onto her rear haunches and peers up at me. But she does it.

"Good girl." Suddenly, she whips her head and ears toward the source of some approaching commotion. Uh oh. It sounds like children—an unpredictable distraction at best—are headed our way. I wonder if I can regain her attention.

"Abbey, wait." This command is more firmly voiced, resulting in the miraculous result of salvaging her attention.

I walk away in a near tip-toe and keep my "stay" hand signal behind me for her to see. This is not a completely legal move in dog obedience, but it's my go-to routine designed as extra insurance. I reach the end-aisle U-turn and glance back. Lo and behold, she sits, waiting for me and avoiding temptation, as a young girl and her older sister round the corner and stop in their tracks at the sight. *Hooray, smart girl.* My heart soars.

"Mommy," the youngest child says, "look." She points a finger toward Abbey and tugs forward, emitting squeals of delight.

I thank the Fates that Mommy is holding the younger child's hand. She slows to lead them down the aisle and around Abbey, who weakly but clearly maintains her sit-stay at my insistent urging. Then they stop right in front of her.

"May they touch her?" the mother asks.

I glance at Arie, who nods, and I say, "Yes, of course." Simultaneously, I release Abbey with an "okay."

86

What an inspiration this dog is today! Abbey allows the children to approach and pet her as they are guided by their mother. The younger child, jumping up and down in tiny leaps, asks if she can hold Abbey's leash, and Abbey allows this transfer while watching me for reassurance. Two minutes later, they move on. Arie is pleased as Abbey doesn't show any fear from this unexpected interaction. It's a good mental and physical pause from our assessment routine, and I'm reminded how important these breaks are from my sometimes too serious expectations. We take a few minutes and frolic together; a game of catching treats, circle right, circle left, feeling our stress levels melt away in this playful connection.

Just a few practice tasks remain on this first formal trip—what I call the "Mom and DAD's Day Out." Arie prepares me for checking out of the store, noting that every task must keep my dog safe and under my attentive, conscious behavior.

The three of us move toward the registers, index cards in hand and ready for purchase. No customers follow me into the checkout line, so I sit Abbey on my left to more easily swipe my card through the machine before seeking Arie's counsel on our next step.

"Place Abbey on your right," she says, "so that other customers don't distract her while you pay for merchandise. That way, she'll be in a safer spot."

I grumble, albeit silently, in protest, scramble to hold my wallet, grab my credit card and shuffle Abbey to my opposite side before dropping two items onto the floor. *How important is this, really?* The clerk smiles as he watches the unfolding scenario. Then another customer enters the line behind me, and the distraction Arie had mentioned becomes obvious when Abbey breaks her stay to sniff and enjoy a new, keenly irresistible encounter. Now understanding the challenges rife at the checkout line, I throw everything down on the register's conveyor belt to quickly move Abbey from my left side to my right. She's finally out of the way, but I must momentarily drop her lead in order to free my hands. This works. The transaction completed, I thank my lucky stars that Abbey kept her stay before sweeping her toward the exit door and out into the awaiting sunshine.

"Ehhhhh!" Uh oh. I already know what that sound means and reluctantly peek back. Arie stands six feet from me and is still inside the foyer.

Huh? Even here?

As if reading my thoughts, Arie nods and smiles.

"When entering or exiting a store with a service dog, remember what I told you? Always wait for outgoing and incoming customers to move past you and Abbey. It keeps her safe and you won't hold up other people who might be intimidated by her."

For someone like me who is always in a rush, learning to eat humble pie isn't going to be easy. But this is a valuable lesson, and I can appreciate the good karma that might come from such mindfulness. Thus, we rewind our exit at these doors for the second time today, finally garnering Arie's approval.

On this first go-round, two customers leaving the store, privy to some of the training taking place, smile with encouragement. Then one asks a question which all DAD and service dog handlers should anticipate.

"What are you training her for?"

My heart jumps at how much to reveal. I weigh my need for privacy with the irrefutable fact that Abbey is with me because she is being trained to perform a needed service, knowing the time has long passed to wish away my condition, as had happened for years in my younger, denial-filled days. Measuring and observing, like always, Arie waits quietly in the background.

Ultimately, I reply, "She's being trained as a service dog—to detect drops in blood sugar."

"That's amazing," comes the response. Mere seconds later, they are gone. I take a deep breath.

Walking out to my car, Arie explains that whether or not to tell people that Abbey is a DAD or a medical alert dog is a personal choice. Not everyone has to know my medical information or the tasks for which we are training her; it's completely up to me. It is then that I realize a simple truth: sometimes revealing information can be a case of sharing too much. Often, less is more. Deciding who to tell and how much to share depends, as always, on the level of trust in your relationships and your need to inform specific people. I know there's no one right approach, and it will take some mental wrestling to figure this out.

I turn on the air conditioning and tell Abbey to jump in. Arie waits while I fasten the safety harness to the seatbelt.

"Can we meet again in a few weeks for more practice?" I ask Arie.

"Sure," she says. "How did you think Abbey did today according to the list?"

Privately, I think nothing about training a DAD seems easy; at least the first time around. But more rational thinking prevails after assessing our session.

"Pretty well. I'm pleased, overall. She didn't seem overwhelmed. We just need more experience."

"I agree," Arie replies, "I'm happy with how well she did. Just get out there with her. Take her to lots of different places. We'll attack a few more PA expectations on the list next time around, okay?"

I nod and scan the car window to check on Abbey. Her chest rises and falls in deep breaths, telling me she's already fallen asleep. I know how drained she feels, because I'm worn out, too.

Waving goodbye, I open the passenger door and plunk a big fat kiss on the top of my sweet girl's head. She nuzzles into me with a deep moan before we finally start toward home, more than ready to cuddle up together for a long and much-needed afternoon's nap.

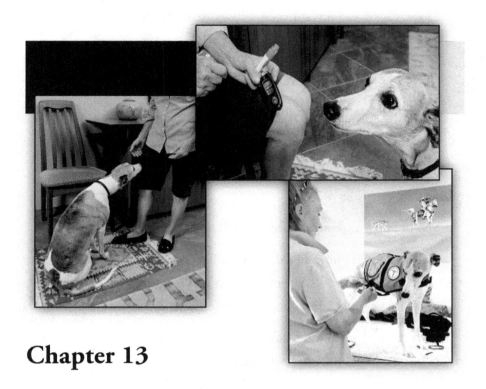

Chapter 13

Eureka! First Independent Alert

Achieving nirvana always seemed out of reach, but I can recall in detail the day Abbey unexpectedly brings it to me. At 2:43 p.m. on September the 18th, as my friend Francie and I wrap up visiting after working on Abbey's service vest measurements and sharing lunch, I stand in her dining room. We are chatting away, trying to finish business but reluctant to end our visit while seven of her regal saluki hounds bark and play in various areas of the house and yard. Abbey is happily ensconced on a nearby chair, triumphantly chewing on one of the salukis' rawhide bones. Midsentence, I sense that something has changed. *What is it?* Something so subtle, it is but a whisper. And then again.

I look down and am stunned. No words come from my mouth.

"Francie," I finally say, "did you see Abbey come up to me?"

"Yes," she replies. "She just got off the chair."

"But Francie, did she touch my leg?"

Francie eyeballs me, trying to understand what I am asking.

I gaze at my heart dog and ask, "What is it? Did you give me a nudge, Abbey?"

She puts her nose to my thigh again, trying to signal me.

I don't quite believe her despite seeing the behavior with my own eyes. She's been prone to give me an alert just to receive praise or a treat. So it usually goes with food-motivated dogs like mine.

"Hmmm," I say, "might as well test my blood sugar to see if she's right. But I really doubt it. I feel fine."

I reach to pull my testing meter out of my carry bag, perch myself on a chair, and set it up on my lap. Abbey stands patiently by my side, quietly waiting. A mere five seconds later on my trusty OneTouch UltraLink meter, the countdown flashes 73. That is low-normal, and I cannot rule out the possibility that my glucose is falling quickly enough to signal Abbey that something is askew. Still, it's not in the danger zone or necessitating any preemptive emergency treatment—not yet, anyway.

I gaze down into her deep, dark brown eyes. *Could she be right?*

I still feel fine. No shaking. No sign of any impending emergency. But the possibility that Abbey senses what I yet cannot pushes me to believe what she is trying to tell me and reward her, just in case my meter and I are wrong.

"Good girl!" I tell her. She happily chows down on a handful of treats before moving away to reclaim her stolen rawhide.

Francie keenly watches both of us as I tuck my testing kit away.

"Did you see that?" I ask Francie, the surprise in my voice seeming to echo in rising rings of sound.

My rhetorical question needs no response, but she nods. I bob my head, unsure, but hope that Abbey is right.

A mere ten minutes later, the shaking sensation in my hands that warns of plummeting blood sugar begins with a hint of thumping heartbeat and jittery sense of desperation. I pop an old salt water taffy fished from a front purse pocket and hard as air-dried clay into my mouth. *Lucky to have this at hand.*

"Francie," I note, "do you realize I'd actually eat this, paper wrapping and all, if I needed to? When your sugar plunges, you'll eat anything to stay alive and conscious. It's a crazy thing."

I smile at Francie and see her eyes open wider as she tries to grasp this statement. *Did I say too much?*

Francie nods, watching me quietly. She's no expert on diabetes, but she understands the struggle it takes to stay well—both emotionally and physically. She's been through her own battles and emerged triumphant. Much like me. We both know the pain of despair and the hard-won gifts of humble hope and gratitude.

On the long ride home from Placitas into Albuquerque, I realize that what Abbey has just done is remarkable, despite the alert being somewhat tenuous, a little too gentle to be easily detected. She signaled me on her own with no verbal prompts and using none of our typically-thawed glucose samples. In a setting on alien turf, surrounded by seven rambunctious salukis, she consciously and independently alerted me to dropping blood sugar. I'd doubted her, believing it was a ploy for a reward. And my doubt had been proven wrong.

Still shivering in disbelief, I pull off the road into a small village center to contact Arie. I'd just read an earlier text asking me to let her know how Abbey does with alerting behaviors over the next few weeks. Ha! This will undoubtedly get a quick response.

> Arie—just coming back from my friend's place in Placitas where I took Abbey to get measured for her service dog vest. My friend has 7 salukis and Abbey wasn't afraid of them! As we were wrapping up, Abbey came up to me and ALERTED ON HER OWN. I thought she just wanted a treat but decided to check my blood sugar. Couldn't believe it because it was 73 but was on the way down. 10 minutes later…58! I'm in heaven.

Within minutes, her reply pings me:

> No sh--! So, this was her first real alert on her own then, right?

My laughter is so piercing, and so nearly on the edge of a vortex of euphoria and disbelief, that its shrillness awakens Abbey from her deep nap. Once started, it doesn't stop. Tears are rolling down my face through waves of convulsive laughter. I know there is so much more to learn, but right now, I don't want to think about anything outside of this astonishing moment. Eureka and nirvana had just intersected in my hands, and it was wildly intoxicating. A miracle? Maybe. But, unquestionably, a breathtaking milestone to be celebrated. Team Abbey is finally moving into new territory, and our future—whatever that looks like--captivates me with its open invitation. The Land of Enchantment, indeed!

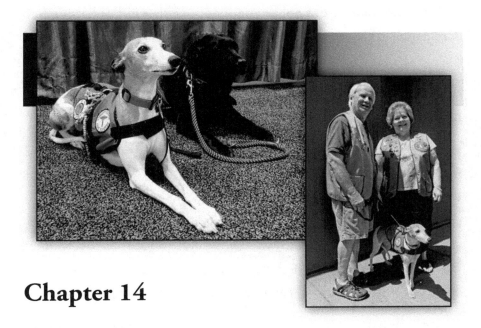

Chapter 14

Positive Advocacy Can Change The World

Not everything goes smoothly when people see a service or medical alert dog in unexpected places. Even their reactions to someone broaching the possibility of bringing along such a dog can be unnerving. It's a situation which surprises most people, exactly because it is largely outside the norm. This is difficult in itself; a world filled with so many people who don't understand. But many are doubters or haters, too; those who don't *want* to understand. Learning how to face these kinds of reactions, with a measure of compassion, is essential to one's well-being and moving normally through day-to-day life when you use a DAD or other type of service dog.

On one afternoon encounter weeks after Abbey's triumphant alert, we return to visit Francie. She shares her perceptions about an Achilles heel in the human-canine service dog world—one I have rarely considered.

"Responsibility for determining how well people understand each other really rests with the handler. The reason problems arise is when handlers only think about their own needs," Francie says.

She continues sharing more of her thinking: that emotional reactions tend to override reason in many situations, whether we are out with our dogs on the agility field, in a rally ring, training obedience or competitively seeking titles like CDX or BOB. This same self-centeredness can kick in when we train and use dogs as DADs or other types of service dogs. We tend to forget that every one of us is emotionally invested in achieving personal goals with our dogs.

As a newcomer to taking my DAD out into the community, I fall right into this same trap; feeling righteously blessed and woefully unprepared for some of the questions hurled my way. When faced with situations that trigger my emotions, I have to admit that I do not feel like a person in control.

Francie tosses me just this type of tidbit to digest on the afternoon of my second visit. "One time," she tells me, "I got on a plane with Tzvi."

Tzvi is Francie's smart-as-all-get-out, pure-Egyptian line saluki, trained as her emotional therapy companion. He's a beautiful soul with a freckled nose bridge and wrapped in a red and white fringed coat. One hundred percent attuned to Francie, he is essential to stabilizing her emotions on a daily basis.

"The flight attendant asked me if I'd like to sit with someone else who also happens to have a service dog. Just because we both had dogs and were on the same flight."

"Hmmm," I mumble, lost for a moment in my own thought wondering what she decided to do. "What did you tell her?"

"I said 'No, thank you.' It was kind of funny, because I felt more than a little surprised that someone else would be on my flight with a service dog. You don't get a lot of that."

For a brief moment, I am baffled, too. There are so many people falsely claiming their dogs are service dogs these days, resulting in escalating tensions and conflicts. I lean in to listen more closely.

She continues, "I sort of thought, the nerve of that person. Someone else actually has a dog, besides me? But I only stayed there, in my head, for a short time."

We both laugh.

"At the end of the flight," Francie says, "I walked up to the woman as we deplaned and asked her how the flight was. You know, to be a good sport."

"What did she say?"

"When I saw her, she signed to me. It was then that I realized she was deaf. It hit me like a freight train. She had every reason and need for her service dog."

Francie adds, "I was really taken aback at my own attitude. How I felt, in a way, more important. I thought only about what I needed— that my dog was so essential to getting me on that plane to fly somewhere. It was the only thing I could think of. Nothing else, and nobody else, mattered right then."

"And?" I prod.

"I realized later after seeing this other woman's real need that it's so important not to judge others. But we all do. Things aren't always what they seem."

Wow," I respond. "That's a gem."

Francie, my new guru of euphemisms in the service dog world, sums up her point.

"It's important not to judge a book by its cover," she says.

I gesture in agreement, thinking what a fitting concept this is when it comes to living with an invisible condition like diabetes. It summarizes my life in all its ups and downs, hopes and fears. I can only aspire to find wisdom in my encounters with people who aggressively doubt my need for having Abbey with me. And my hope to find some measure of grace while learning how much personal information to share with strangers.

I broach my experience of visiting an Albuquerque garden nursery a few months back, still recalling the overwhelming rage that trounced all reason.

"Francie," I begin, "when I was just months into training Abbey, I stopped at a garden center in the Valley to pick up some herbs and vegetables. I'd been there so many times before and saw lots of people taking their dogs in with them. I'd planned to take Abbey in with me, that day, for the first time as a service dog in training.

Francie raised her red-tinged eyebrows in anticipation.

"I got out of the car with Abbey on a lead. Then I saw a sign hanging on the garden gate."

"Yeah?" she asks. "What did it say?"

I shake my head, remembering my reaction. "It said: 'No dogs allowed, except for task-performing service dogs.' I thought about you and Tzvi. How people working there might keep you from going in. That really upset me, because you need him."

Francie nods. I rush to present my argument; a tirade of emotion, even now.

"What about returning veterans with post-traumatic stress disorders, for example? You hear a lot about them being helped by service dogs. They're emotional support animals, and many vets really need their dogs to function. The ADA law shouldn't exclude that kind of help from anyone."

"Well, it does," Francie says quietly. "No emotional support dogs are technically allowed. They're not considered to be service dogs because they're not trained to do a specific, physical task. But I bring Tzvi almost everywhere I go because, well, you're right. He balances me. Keeps me on the straight and narrow. He's so well-trained that there are never too many questions. I have appropriate papers to show if anyone challenges me, and it always works out okay."

I glance across the room at the handsome Tzvi, lolling on his plush southwestern bed that Francie lovingly sewed. He's oblivious to my percolating crusade on his behalf.

"You'll learn more as you go along," Francie replies. "Tell me what happened next. Did you take Abbey in with you?"

My breath comes more rapidly.

"I was so upset at this injustice and the words on that sign that my heart started hammering. I couldn't even think clearly. So I just wandered inside the gate and left Abbey with Bob in the entryway."

"You didn't have to do that," Francie says.

"I know. I tried to push away my anger while I picked up a few plants, but I put them all back. By then, I was too upset to buy anything and realized it was important to talk this over with the owner."

"Did you?" she asks, watching me carefully.

"Yep. I went inside and asked to speak to someone in charge, but neither the owner or manager were there. I'm sorry to say that I totally lost it. I laid into the gal at the register and yelled at her that their sign was illegal. That it made no sense. That I had shopped there for years, but if they didn't change the policy, I wouldn't be back."

Francie regards me with the same expression I often get from my husband; a *calm down and think logically* look. I wait for her impending admonishment.

"Well," Francie notes, right on cue, "you get more flies with honey than vinegar. They must have had a good reason to put out that sign. Like dogs peeing on their plants or eating and destroying lots of the plants, don't you think?"

I return a face that is surprised and more. Anger wraps its tentacles around my reply.

"Really? You think that's *right?"*

Embarrassed now at having to admit the extent of my reaction, my tone drops. "I ended up screaming in frustration. That gal must have thought I was a nutcase."

"You'll see," Francie says. "You were just starting to train Abbey, and you ran into an obstacle that offended you. There will be lots more of them."

My eyebrows lift again in disbelief. Mostly that she sides with the business, but in part, because she's so calm in the face of my churning emotions. I'm not sure why she doesn't understand what I just related to her. The unfairness of it seems so palpable, my voice shakes describing the experience.

"Remember," Francie coaches, "there's so much that people don't understand. You know the law, but our job is to represent our dogs and make life easier for *everyone* with a service dog. Lots of people ruin it for others by being angry, lecturing or even pretending their pets are service dogs when they're not."

Somehow, I begin to grasp a snippet of what my friend is saying: that being a positive ambassador rather than a lawsuit-threatening aggressor works magic to win supporters. This is hard to hear and even tougher to assimilate.

I am just beginning to fathom that the road Team Abbey is traveling, while it sometimes detours into hostile territory, beckons us toward a different kind of experience. Despite some emotional ups and downs, it is essential that I learn how to manage questions and attitudes that shake my personal boundaries and move me to a higher plane of understanding. This quest promises as much meaning as any dog title I could have previously imagined before embarking on this path.

Some days, I find myself nearly trembling, much like my impatient whippets, ready to fly toward the lure that dangles in front of us. Like them, I can sense the tingling agony of a 'wait!' command and see them straining to hear their secret release word, telling them they can finally move forward. I can almost see, from Abbey's eyes, just how rocky that balance is. So many repetitions. An overflow of wait-and-sees. I feel it, too, sitting on this cusp, so close to being a successful DAD team. But I know, just like with the hyper-focused attention demanded by canine pursuits like rally, agility and obedience training, it is all about taking time to tweak the commands that help train us in needed behaviors that move us forward—releasing us only when we've become a solid team. Only then will Abbey and I be able to promote our work, and all its wondrous possibilities, in the community.

These days, I hear my meta-coaching voice—a sort of mantra—more and more, saying: You go, girl! Keep putting one foot in front of the other! This helps me nix any self-doubts so that I can wrap myself in newfound confidence and a growing sense of accountability. Teetering on the brink of success, I realize that all good things will come in time. Making a difference and being secure enough to look outside myself is what this journey is ultimately all about. Just a few more essential steps, and we are nearly there.

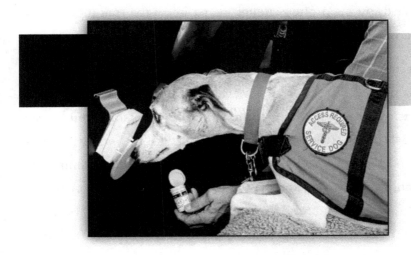

Chapter 15

Teaming To Train The Difficult Car Alert

There are parts of training a DAD that would be much easier to pretend were unneeded. Required behaviors you wish were just plain optional. One of my most dreaded tasks has turned out to be figuring out how to move Abbey's nose touch of the door chime to a new setting: triggering it as an alert in my car. That's right; picture it— the car alert, with my dog behind me, and me a seat away.

I'd had no difficulty whatsoever training Abbey to alert to my low glucose levels while indoors. But the mere thought of how to reach and teach her while driving, and for all intents and purposes a field away, gives me hair-raising heebie-jeebies. What is it about training her to alert in a different location which triggers my wildest fears? It all makes me so squirrely that I've pushed this DAD task late into our training cycle. Truthfully, it was almost forgotten except, of course, for my nagging conscience which intractably refused to let it disappear. The thought has tag-touched my brain often enough that I knew the training for a car alert had to eventually take place.

The self-imposed week to confront my concerns finally arrives, trapping me in a "this is it" moment. It feels like the much-dreaded annual arrival of our high desert phenomenon; amassing tumbleweeds spinning into maelstroms on the backs of biting spring winds, with me and my poor dogs, whether on an agility field or walking community trails, caught in their vortices. We have found ourselves hoping, and indeed lucky, to remain upright on the blusteriest of these days. Yep; it is a close enough match to say that my dread feels just like the onslaught of these southwestern squalls. But I summon my resolve, propelled in part by guilt, and throw myself into the task.

To better understand how to train Abbey, I reread Martinez and Barns' words and wait for any glimmer of light. *Help. Me. Picture. This.* I chant the refrain ever so precisely, squinting my eyes to capture how to put it all together and seek good karma from my dedicated efforts. Still struggling and in near desperation, I move back a chapter to material already covered and begin picturing the alert chain as described. I jot a few notes to try these steps over the next several weeks, finally relaxing at the ease with which images come to me.

I stop here, knowing that this part of Abbey's DAD training requires careful attention to each detail in the process of succeeding with a workable car alert. Paper and pen in hand, I painstakingly summarize the first few steps in a "cheat sheet" meant to guide me through the sequence. All that remains is pulling together the needed supplies.

This task has its challenges, too. Despite practicing low glucose alerts with the doggie door chime Pebble Smart since its arrival four months earlier, I still face the challenge of trying to find a way to mount it onto a board of some type that will be stable enough for Abbey to nose it in the car. What to use and where to place the chime in the car are technical questions that lack technical answers.

I make a mental note: this calls for a formal consultation with my engineer husband whose ideas are always practical, albeit quite different, from my own creative take. I compromise on the initial trial run to test the workability of his idea—anchoring the bell chime with screws onto a folded metal piece designed to slide into the lower window frame behind me. Might this damage the rubber molding or cause the passenger door to loosen and break when it opens? Despite thinking that my own ideas might yield better results than my husband's, I acquiesce in the interest of equality and a firm belief in the value of testing all possible ideas. And thus, phase one commences.

My doubts over the test design go unfounded through the first weeks of training. The chime stays put, and it works well with the receiver placed nearby in one of the front seat cup holders so that the "nose button" transmitter can successfully trigger the bell. Except for minor modifications, the prototype for attaching the doggie doorbell is a success. Another humble pie moment? Not really. All that really matters is moving forward and getting the job done. By tackling my partner's design ideas and finding success, I get to accrue many points in the tally sheet of our relationship.

Despite the realization of the doggie doorbell design, the hoped-for celebration is still a long way off. There is much to do: finding mutual times to train with a helper and setting up formal training dates for car-alert sessions that don't get nixed because one of us is too busy or too tired after returning home from work. Managing time issues to conduct these training sessions is a surprisingly challenging component. There are many days when the dog is too dog-tired to pay attention, and my plans for training have to be scrapped. Three players in the training mix (my husband, dog and me) is a lot like letting dogs loose on a field; each one moving pell-mell or dropping from exhaustion in response to different drives.

One such session unfolds ominously on a weeknight. Bob and I rendezvous at the house, intent on fitting one little car-alert session into the last remnants of light. With no time to grab dinner, we rush into the training fray and lead our hungry, sleepy dog into the back passenger seat, hoping for victory. "Hope" turns out to be the operative word.

I *hope* the sequence I picture includes any behavior from our DAD that resembles a car alert.

I *hope* to give the dog treats but am unsure who should give a reward when needed—me in the driver's seat or Bob sitting alongside Abbey.

I *hope* we'll finish before all light leaves the sky.

Without enough energy to follow through on training Abbey, this session is doomed to fail. All Abbey gives us tonight mirrors our own limited attention spans. If nothing else, it reminds me about the critical nature of timing.

The next round of car alert training is scheduled on a weekend when there is still light in the late afternoon sky. We are not quite so tired and are bathed in the luxury of a few days off from work when I remind Bob that one important task awaits. At that, we guide Abbey to the car, one of us fueled by Thin Mint Girl Scout cookies, the other by a few bites of guacamole-laden chips, as I command her to jump into the passenger seat.

This session seems different from the last fiasco. Abbey is alert. She jumps up into the car in anticipation of tackling something fun. Somehow, so do we. And that's how it goes.

In the car, Abbey waits expectantly. Each of us hold treats, ready to reinforce just about any behavior resembling a car alert. I climb into the driver's seat while Bob slips into the back next to the dog.

"Ready?" I ask. This rhetorical question is more for my own benefit than for anyone else. The receiver sits beside me on the middle console with the doggie chime hanging on the passenger window nearest Abbey. I glance in my rearview mirror and adjust it, the better to see my spouse and to observe my dog who has no clue what is about to unfold, except for the promise of an awaiting treat-fest. *Please let this work.*

Bob nods. "Roger," he signals in typical engineer geek-talk.

At that, I pop open my scent sample as quietly as possible and steal a glance in the mirror. I can't see Abbey well, so I twist my body to get a better view. She is oblivious to our purpose for the set-up. She sits and waits for me to start up the car and take her somewhere, anywhere, fun. But she doesn't alert me by ringing the bell.

"Jeesh," I mutter. *Fine, maybe this isn't the time to be subtle.*

My training partner tries to temper my frustration by prompting her. "Abbey," he coaches, just like he's heard me say a hundred times, "What is it?"

I hold my breath. Will she make a connection between the scent, the trigger question typically asked that cues her to check on her olfactory capture of low blood sugar, and the nearby bell?

Like me, I know Bob is worried she won't get it. He jumps in and, again, tries assisting Abbey in connecting the dots.

"Abbey, look." He points to the sample and then the bell, all while holding a treat in his fingers. There is no doubt she wants that treat. I know this because her nose pokes at Bob's hand and works heroically to convince him to release it. To his credit, he holds on tight.

I'm reminded that aging is not for the timid as I twist further toward her from the driver's seat with the open canister of low glucose scent, causing my neck and back to spasm. Suddenly, just as objections begin to form in my head and defeat signals me to raise a white flag, Abbey rings the bell, as she should, since the scent sample is essentially in her face.

Bob and I both smile and shout out verbal markers for her success. My back twinges are momentarily forgotten in the euphoria.

"Yes!" I sing out, over and over, like a glitched recording. "Yes, yes, yes!"

"Good girl, Abbey! Ring the bell." Bob's head nods. His finger points. His eyes crinkle with pride.

My brain thunders. *Will she be a one-hit wonder? Or will she repeat the sequence?* How I fervently hope it is a strong building block to understanding and performing the essential car alert.

The bell rings again and again before these doubts escape my lips. There is no discounting the fact that the sample scent has reached Abbey, helping her know what she needs to do.

Ding, dong! Ding, dong! Ding, dong!

I laugh. Bob joins in.

The treats spill out of my helper's hands while my own verbal markers recognize Abbey's correct learning efforts.

"Yes, Abbey, yes!"

Never mind that I am waving the sample scent all around me like a conductor entreating a crescendo from musicians. I am merely grateful that the car alert seems to have been connected to the appropriate scent and behavior. Realizing the impact of all the body contortions needed to teach Abbey the car alert, it dawns on me that it's time to rest and call it a day.

The three of us wrap up our session in the parked car. It was a bit too long and a lot too obvious shoving the scent dramatically through the air. But it is a solid start for the remaining car alert trainings to come, some of them still to be arranged in a "moving" vehicle.

"When can we try this again?" I ask Bob. He shrugs, pats me on the shoulder and leads Abbey inside, leaving me to figure out the specifics for the next session. Everything in its own time, I remind myself. I'm tired. We all are. The epiphanies that come, after following so many necessary training recommendations, are draining. They take commitment. But I realize that the process works if one is able to fully pledge time to it.

When I head back inside, twilight has fallen. I am more than ready to rest and contemplate the implications of tonight's training session. After all, it is a weekend. What better time is there to celebrate and rejoice in the small steps we just made? Yes, there's more to do. There's always more to do. But knowing my canine teammate is learning to be there for me, doing her new job to help me manage mine, is worth every minute spent building the bridge we want to cross.

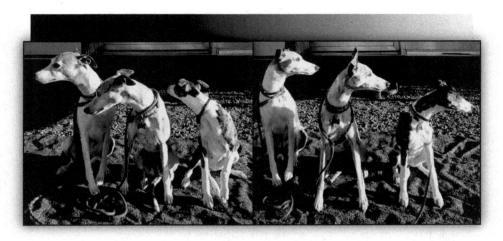

Chapter 16

Bloopers: The Good, The Bad & The Ugly

Quirks and bloopers come in all shapes and sizes. And lest my ego grow too intolerable at our stacking successes, I'll admit that Abbey and I make plenty of mistakes traveling the training highway.

Some are humbling. One day, I meet a colleague at a popular café and end up being scolded by the observant wait-staff when I place an order for Abbey's plate of food on the floor.

"We don't let pets eat off customer plates. Here, use this instead," an anonymous server swoops in to say while handing me a paper plate. Then my friend chimes in. "It's okay. Don't worry, Kathy. We all learn something every day." I shrug in agreement, acknowledging my friend's gentle statement, while chastising myself. Of course, the waitress is probably right, too, but I am too embarrassed to process her comments. All I have as evidence of the need for further reflection is my face burning the color of crimson.

When I recount the mistakes made on this outing to my mentor Francie, she says, "Don't anthropomorphize. Remember, a working dog has a job to do, and she's not going to die of hunger because she skips a snack or a meal." That pushes me to swallow a small slice of humble pie and reflect on its unexpected benefits—stretching my understanding by mulling and accepting the supportive advice of a friend who once walked in my new shoes. I slowly realize that the simple truths governing proper public behavior for service dogs, and how to elicit them, give me a deeper understanding of the human-dog relationship. How can I help but learn from stepping into all the slip-ups which inevitably generate such unusual opportunities for personal growth?

Nothing seems more important than this—except maybe holding onto a sense of humor. That restaurant scene, fueled by my lack of attention in understanding my dog's role, along with the finer points of restaurant etiquette for service dogs, is one memory that still generates convulsive laughter well after the café incident.

Food is always a conundrum—in all its temptations and constraints. Rarely is a day spent in a training session unaccompanied by treats to bolster behaviors Abbey must master. But out in public, and even at home, the irony of such a high value placed on a service dog or DAD *ignoring* the temptation of smells and foods does not escape me. Trips to grocers, plant nurseries and restaurants are met by a barrage of aromas followed by my dog's all-too-willing embrace of yet another opportunity for a delightful sensory field trip. Teaching her to ignore the temptation of food dropped by others or placed on countertops for visitors demands my constant attention. The number of apologies I make for her innumerable cunning scarfings? Countless, and all of them, priceless. Each incident forces me to think like a dog, all the better to understand the lure of the dark side.

Well beyond humbling are the oversights sometimes made in the DAD training process. I wrestle with the fact that these can be considered life-threatening if left unaddressed. The time of greatest concern is nighttime—when I most need to rely on Abbey to alert me at her drowsiest. Rigging the doggie doorbell on my nightstand, keeping treats filled to overflowing in a nearby container to reward alerts; it all requires nonstop training. There are times I fuss over her reluctance to awaken. "She's so lazy" is my usual comment on good nights where drops in glucose happen but don't necessarily scare me. Other nights, I cry in frustration as I wonder when I will be able to depend on my DAD completely. In reality, the blooper is, in large part, me; not wanting to stay up for hours or get up in the middle of the night for a training session. Though the humor is often lean and challenging for me to grasp in these nighttime situations, it's still there.

These are necessary reality checks. It takes constant work to admit these gaffes, redouble my efforts at training Abbey toward better accuracy, and work on shaping and sharing my dog's best public "face"—seen by others as Abbey having extraordinary training and manners. Beyond these sessions, reinforcing specific DAD behaviors folds an additional element into our days. Admittedly, there are times I want to give up, chiefly when every mistake we make as a team snakes its way into new layers of humility at levels I didn't think possible.

More than once in a while, though, a blooper brings insight. A reason to keep moving forward, learn, reflect, shrug off mistakes or sense of blame, and find an opportunity to laugh, affirming that the path I've chosen is indeed worthwhile. This next episode is one of them: the day I bring Abbey to Staples to once again meet our trainer for a practice Public Behavior Access Test run-through.

On a sizzling summer morning, Abbey and I creep down the aisle at Staples for our second outing with Arie, who walks behind, coaching us. I want it all to go so well. *Please don't let the pressure I'm feeling creep down Abbey's lead.* I know, from handling Abbey in the show ring, that a handler's emotions are sensed by one's dog, and that doubt often leads to a self-fulfilling prophesy; one where the dog doesn't perform well because the command is sabotaged by fear. As if I need any confirmation, Abbey looks up with her piercing eyes, trying to ascertain more clues from my body language so she can do what I want. *Stay in the moment.* I take a deep breath followed by another.

"Let's move to another aisle toward some shoppers. I want you to go through merchandise on a few shelves and get Abbey to stay put while you step away from her."

I nod. *Move forward. Just do it.* I paste a smile on my face and start the sequence of movement toward a nearby customer, remembering to slow Abbey to a near stop as we approach the end of the aisle. This is needed for her safety—a quick check that she won't be confronted by something unexpected coming around a corner.

"C'mon, girl, turn right." I begin to relax as she follows suit. We move as if in slow motion around another corner and approach a shopper scanning merchandise.

"All right, Abs," I say. "Sit." I glance at Arie for more direction.

"Let's put Abbey in a sit-stay and you can move away from her to pick things up off shelves. Stand on her lead to make sure she doesn't wander, but try to keep her in place to give her practice waiting for you, okay?"

I take a deep breath to process this multi-faceted request, hoping there are no distractions.

"Okay." Another breath pushes me into action. There's no turning back now.

"Come, girl, right here." I motion Abbey to swing around me. "Sit," I say. "Now, stay." My hand moves in front of her face. Extra reassurance that she'll obey the hand-signaled command, if not my verbal direction.

She moves and interprets like an old soul: calmly, obediently, effortlessly gliding into place. Then she sits, watching. My heart swells.

"Good girl," I say, kissing the top of her soft, brindle head before stepping away and moving down the aisle a few feet, pretending to examine different merchandise. Abbey stays where she is, despite the slight rustling of calendars and notebooks by the nearby shopper.

I smile and chance glancing away for just a few seconds from Abbey toward Arie. Then I take a few steps to pretend-shop another item.

An unknown temptation pulls Abbey to the customer we passed just moments before. The woman is dressed in a simple skirt and jacket. A big, black, multi-sectioned purse hangs off her right shoulder, completely open. She seems oblivious to us.

Warning signals buzz me to be aware. I pull tighter on Abbey's lead as we follow Arie's request to move on by, even as Abbey strains. I hold tight, roping her in, as the stranger bends down to reach through calendars on the bottom shelf. *How can she not hear us or sense that we're right here?* I can't imagine how she is ignoring this commotion and shake my head, disbelieving the possibility.

But Abbey, for one, is definitely not unaware. Quite the opposite, she's hyper-aware, which is par for a sighthound. *Touché. Hey—no need right now for that dry sense of humor. Pay attention.* Now appropriately self-redirected, I grasp what my dog sees: an invitation. The woman's bag looms right in front of my curious beast-in-training. It lures her like a fish to bait, and in the next moment, Abbey's long twitching nose dives gently but deep into the abyss as I watch in a frozen state of mixed humor and horror. *Ah—the crux of comedies.*

"Abbey, no," I command in the most authoritarian voice I can muster. "Here. By my side," I say sternly, mostly for our trainer's benefit.

I hope Arie missed what just happened. I tug my dog to me, placing her back in heel position. I want to laugh, but instead I'm in limbo, watching the customer move down the aisle, unaware of the transgression we just committed. I bend down to commiserate with Abbey, trying not to laugh at her keen observational powers and stealth. Be the model trainer, I admonish myself. And then my eyes meet my trainer's. Arie stands at the end of the aisle, a look of hilarity on her face. She has seen it all. She raises her hands indicating a stalemate. We both laugh heartily, and I can't help but fall in love with this moment.

On my way home, I begin to visualize what *might* have happened if Abbey's doggie behaviors had ramped into no-no territory. My imagination cannot clear one offbeat image from all the possible "what ifs," and I lean over the steering wheel, gasping, tears rolling down my cheeks at the sheer craziness of the idea. What if Abbey's precious hound-scenter of a nose had gravitated to that stranger's crotch and not just into her open purse? It could happen. For me, it's just three degrees of separation from the saying "could've, would've, should've"—and much too close for comfort.

It's no minor take-away that the giddiness, complexities and epiphanies of bloopers on this day, and others like it, delight me. I love this journey and the intricacies required by Abbey and me as a team moving in and out of public life, weaving our way from one scenario to the next. Challenges come in many forms, all of them interesting, but it's ironic how trivial thoughts like this can foster gratitude from even the tiniest of life's lessons. I'm so thankful for this humor on such a serious journey. There are so many laughs in the goof-ups, if only we allow them to lighten our load.

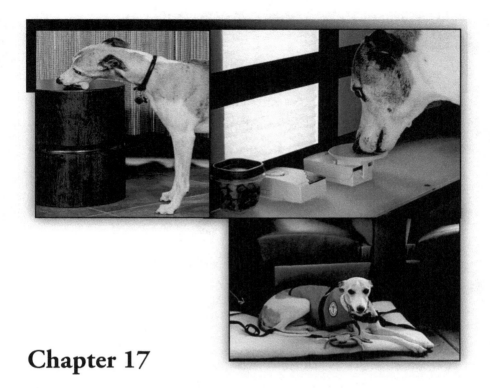

Chapter 17

The 24/7 Quest To Generalize DAD Alerts

On a glorious, sun-warmed early September day where cotton swaths of cumulous clouds dance across impossibly blue skies and the last of the monarch butterflies and bees flit around gold-buttoned santolina, I'm reminded of just how beautiful New Mexico really is and how lucky I am to live here. The spaces around me are vast and open; the hardiest of the remaining frilly hollyhocks still bloom and smells of the first roasted chile crop waft in the air—nature's gifts of comfort and glory before the coming cold and dark of winter. My phone rings and I answer it only to hear my soul sister and dear friend Jules' agitated voice. She also lives with Type 1 and has endured for one year longer than me—which is to say seemingly forever.

Something isn't right. I reluctantly break with a feeling of harmony to find out what's wrong.

"Kat, I've been trying to reach you—a terrible thing has happened," she says all in one breath. Her voice cracks and then fades. I can tell that she can barely bring herself to reveal more; Jules and I have known each other for decades, and we've never lacked an opportunity to talk and share our feelings—especially about the ups and downs of living with this diabetes.

"What is it, Jules? What's wrong?" I say.

"I don't know how to tell you this. It's just awful."

I remain quiet, waiting.

"It's DuLea. From camp."

I can't imagine what Jules has to say. We had just spent an exhilarating week with DuLea and other campers while running the activity program for the ADA's New Mexico summer diabetes camp on the grounds of Camp Stoney in Santa Fe. With so many returning campers and staff, the camaraderie of eight weeks ago still wraps me in jubilation. What could be so awful? I breathe deeply trying to maintain an even keel.

"Jules, what has happened? Is she in the hospital?"

"No," Jules replies, her voice dropping so low that I have to strain to hear her. "Sh-she died. In her sleep."

I shake my head and sit down hard on a nearby chair.

"Jules, she's just eleven. How could this have even happened? *What do you mean?*" My voice rises in disbelief and anger at the unjustness of such an event. I love this girl with her infectious in-love-with-life nature. Denial swoops in.

"It's impossible," I retort. "How do you even know this happened?"

"One of the counselors called to tell me. She said DuLea went to bed a few nights ago and got up to eat something because she had a headache and her blood sugar was low," Jules says.

"Oh no."

"Her mom found her in the morning. She had fallen out of bed or something. And...and...they tried...but they couldn't save her. They called for an ambulance but it was too late to do anything."

Jules' voice cracks as my mind whirls in and out of dark emotions; the utter sense of betrayal and hopelessness waiting to consume us. My eyes flood. Searing pain creeps from my right forehead across my skull.

I try to picture the unbelievable scene and feel only horror. How will those of us touched by this sweet, amazingly vibrant girl ever be able to grapple with or accept this news?

"Jules," I finally say, "when is the funeral?"

"I'll find out," Jules replies.

"All right. Thank you. Let's plan on meeting there, Jules. I can't be there without you."

"I know, Kat. I feel terrible. We'll be there for each other, okay?"

"Love you, Jules," I say.

Days later, I move slowly as I pull on pants and a top for DuLea's service. Every piece of me wants to scream "no", but I push forward. I meet Jules just outside the Mt. Calvary sanctuary in Albuquerque. We grab hands and hug tightly in the harsh heat, finally releasing each other. We are both afraid to walk inside and see DuLea's relatives, but we agree to spend a few moments there and try to share our grief and love for this amazing girl. Our young friend lays dressed in her Sunday finest that too easily might have served her at a party or camp dance. She appears as beautiful as always. Jules and I approach her family and then move in ever so gently to share our goodbyes and love. The worst is yet to come; moving to our young friend's graveside gathering and burial.

"I cannot believe this," I say to Jules. My voice breaks and my throat gulps for air, but there is none to be found on such a morose day when substantial humidity hangs like a weighty curtain of grief.

"It could happen to us. To any of us. At any time," I say, picturing all the friends we know and love from our camp family. Tears stream down my face, prompting Jules to sob.

Jules reaches to squeeze me again, as we move reluctantly with DuLea's family—a small group hushed to near-silence—to a prepared plot that holds a pristine white casket accented in gold decorative touches on each corner. Thankful to see that it is finally closed, Jules and I stand shoulder to shoulder behind the small rows of seats, compelled to bear witness to the life and loss of our sweet DuLea.

When the minister finishes speaking, Jules and I back away. It hurts too much to watch DuLea's casket being lowered into the ground. Nor can we bear the thought of gathering back at the family home. Once away from earshot and in range of our vehicles parked nearby, we do the only thing we can that doesn't require words or questions: we sit down on the ground and weep until waves of hurt and fear tumble free.

Heartbroken soul sisters inconsolable at the raw loss that is altogether too close.

It is only decades later with the onset of so much supportive technology in diabetes management tools, and the possibility of getting meaningful alerts from a well-trained DAD, that I can envision another very different ending to this tragedy. I'll always wish the outcome was different, and better, for DuLea and her family.

DuLea's presence in my life remains a strong catalyst for the connections I make and the work I do with others in the world of diabetes. She is one of the reasons that Team Abbey is here at all. Losing DuLea provides me with a formidable reminder of the work I've yet to accomplish with my own dog.

The behavior alerts performed by a DAD cannot be overstated as being too essential to keeping one's physical and mental health in balance. Despite admitting to an occasional streak of laziness and wanting to skip a day of training my own dog, I am reminded of Martinez and Barns' rationale which minces no words, stating: "a poorly trained DAD is as bad as having no DAD at all."

This is precisely what I fear and what drives me forward. I need to count on both Abbey and the technical equipment that help me manage my diabetes to keep me healthy and happy. In the Abbey-DAD Department, she is still struggling to master giving the much-needed nighttime alert for my habitually plummeting blood sugars.Being roused to treat "lows" with a simple source of glucose is essential in order to avoid trips to the ER or worse. This is why being able to count on getting these trained alerts is a 24/7 job for a DAD and my unequivocal expectation of Abbey—every time it's needed; every place we are. It is the literal definition of DAD team success in the realm of living with diabetes.

My attempts to tip the scale in our favor start with readdressing our nighttime nemesis. For months, I have grappled with why Abbey is not waking me when necessary during sleep, in spite of her clear mastery of low blood sugar alerts. Is it a breed-related trait? Could sleeping with her pack be so comforting that it dulls her sensory abilities and overrides her training? I wrack my brain, digging into reasons and possible solutions, entertaining any changes in my thinking that might provide a training path forward to overcome a potential disaster.

A recent scenario unfolds in my mind as I explore this riddle. Abbey and I crawl into bed late at night, and her deep desire to be with her pack is obvious by her audible claim to me as she snuggles close. I review my routine nighttime checklist before I can consider turning off the light.

Don't lay down yet: check your glucose level.

But it's so late and I'm really tired. Can't I just skip this one night?

The possibility is tempting, but as I gaze at Abbey, already lost in dreams, I wonder if she will awaken me if needed.

Naw, that's not a good idea now, is it? What if she sleeps through your crash? C'mon now, don't risk it.

More what-ifs start piling up. With my brain recharging, the improbability of sleep looms. I disentangle Abbey from my armpit, where her nose pushes ever deeper into my softest pillow, while I head out to work on my computer.

A short time later, I move back to the bedroom. The house is quiet except for chainsaw snores coming from Bob, who has again neglected to switch on his CPAP before falling into a near-dead sleep. The raw, guttural noises don't seem to impede the dogs' slumber. I laugh, thinking that Bob's rough breathing must be some sort of musical fodder to the dogs. Abbey opens one eye as I enter the room, then nestles closer to her man and groans back into blissful oblivion.

Hurry up, you need some sleep.

Don't forget to test your blood sugar.

I'd like to forget that obligation at this late hour. But I heed my own reminder with a sigh.

Five, four, three, two, one. I silently count down with the meter, wishing I had my CGM—now on order—so that this could all go much faster.

Uh oh. Can't go to sleep on a blood sugar like that.

The meter reads 69. Not so low that it poses an immediate danger, but too close to dropping lower to be able to slip under the covers and get some sleep just yet.

Then I observe my dog. Yes, that dog, the trained one. She is sound asleep, her four limbs outstretched and pumping away in indescribable pleasure while she yips, ever so slightly, at some roadrunner or jackrabbit running through her dreams.

"Abbey?" I call, mindful of not wanting to miss an in-the-moment training opportunity.

She moans and scrunches closer to Bob. Her eyes are still closed.

I try again. "Abbey, help. Help Mommy."

We have trained with sample scents of glucose levels in the mid-60s and lower, but this one seems close enough that she might awaken and give me an alert. Instead, her long nose nudges three times into the soft, clean-scented sheets, like she's digging deeper into her dream.

Lordy, what good are you? I am miffed and call her name again. The alpha sleeps—oblivious to my dream-crasher of a call.

Doggonit. I give up and throw off the bedcovers, padding barefoot on the earth-colored saltillo tiles to the kitchen. I crack the refrigerator door, scouring for some tasty morsel that will both satisfy and hold me steady through the night. Ahh, that's it: peanut butter and blackberry jam. Happy with my choice, I remove the jars from the refrigerator, place them on the counter, and then open the lids for my poised spoon to dig right in.

A soft sound moves in my direction. Abbey stands there watching. Waiting.

I roll my eyes in disbelief. Really? *The trained DAD who wouldn't awaken at my request or alert to my dropping glucose actually stands before me?*

Making an appearance in response to the fridge door opening, no doubt. Oh, but to be a neuron in that brain. Or the omniscient creator of canines. Even a dog psychologist or vet. ANYTHING to better understand what makes a dog tick and gives the average person insight to canine thinking and behavior.

Abbey tilts her head, now fully observant.

"What is it?" I ask, the palms of my hands lifted upward. It's our given question that, used routinely, triggers her to signal an alert if needed. She moves toward me, only then, and nudges my leg in a formal alert behavior.

"Good girl!" I respond, and sigh, before rewarding her with a small treat before we both head back to bed.

This same situation plays out several times each month. Abbey's current behavior is the antagonist to the protagonist needed in this mystery which, to solve, requires my best thinking, some faith and more training sessions. Changing up the timing of our "nighttime alert" training sessions might make a significant difference by moving my expectations of her to alert from a deep state of sleep to early morning hours. Resolutions that address increased reliability from my dog continue, but some level of worry, on my part, remains.

Living long-term with diabetes, and losing a number of friends to low blood sugar crashes over the years, I can't help but think about how crucial this nighttime alert is to survival. It is such a vital issue that I identify two behaviors for backup alert training—each meant to make a difference in getting help when my blood sugar is too low to easily help myself.

The first one is a "third party alert"—also known as a TPA. This is the process of training canines to enact a chain of communication about an emergency. Watching my dog give me typical alerts for low glucose levels but seeing that there is nothing else in place for her to let other people know about emergencies helps me realize the importance of TPAs. And following this realization, I think: *Who better to share the 'low blood sugar alert' with than my lucky husband?* With this goal in mind, the TPA training has begun and is nearly mastered.

A second lifesaving behavior evolves from my hope to get more help from my DAD than a mere notification that my blood sugar is dropping. Abbey's trained nudges to my leg and touches to my hand, though certainly helpful, lack the extra assistance I've wished for and needed more than once. The answer comes to me as I observe her working: Why can't Abbey be trained to recognize, find and bring me some type of glucose in a pending emergency? This is how the retrieval of glucose tablets becomes part of our team's repertoire. It's a fun behavior to train in the scheme of alert behaviors for a DAD—not to mention being handy, useful and capable of engendering heaps of gratitude! My dog likes this, particularly because she knows that my appreciation is almost always translated into a language she understands; praise and treats galore. We simultaneously continue training and making progress on our nighttime alerts. In the world of managing the highs and lows of ever-changing blood sugar levels, the peace of mind gained 24/7 from using these training techniques, in combination with insulin pump and CGM technology, is a priceless asset.

There are many times when I think about how diabetes has so deeply touched me in ways both good and bad. On the good days, I am like anyone else and feel invincible; able to fling myself with joy into all the things I love, set new goals and move forward with faith and confidence. On days that are bleaker, I hug Abbey a bit closer and seek her companionship which somehow lets me breathe a bit easier. Sometimes, memories of all the people I've loved, and some dear ones I've lost like Rick and DuLea, come rushing in. Those are the days when Abbey senses my emotions and lifts her face to mine, licking tears that run in rivers down my cheeks, until the feelings pass and the world is right again.

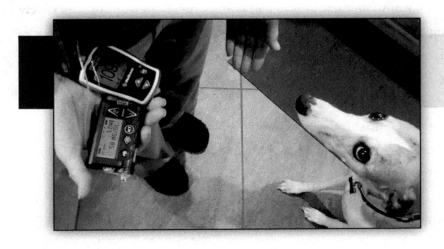

Chapter 18

Sometimes The Dog Is Smarter

If there is one situation dreaded by everyone trying to manage their diabetes and stay out of trouble, it's failure. In the world of living with diabetes, this means one issue with enormous implications: equipment malfunction. Most everyone living with this condition has felt the surging grip of adrenaline followed by denial dwindling to feelings of resignation and disappointment when problems happen; pump sets stay in too long for insulin to remain effective or batteries run dry or Continuous Glucose Monitors shriek alerts. Choice words, exploding tempers, scrambling to circumvent potential disaster by calling a family member or friend for intervention: none of these methods immediately alter the reality of our heavy reliance on the consistent operation of technology to run our programs and keep diabetes-related crises in the background of our daily lives.

One of these situations strikes home when I am working obsessively long hours in an all-out "I can do everything best" model teacher mode. I face a deadline of eight days to prepare more than three weeks' intensive instruction for my gifted third, fourth and fifth graders. On top of this goal comes grading and then filling out lengthy student progress reports to share with my twenty students and their parents for upcoming formal conferences scheduled prior to leaving the country on a several-weeks-long Fulbright trip. The pressure is high. The stress level, extraordinary. The opportunity to set priorities, moot. Everything in this community of high expectations—deservedly so in any school— has to be tackled; nothing can be left unfinished or unplanned. I am determined, with my eye on the prize, to wrap up everything before my substitute steps into my shoes and professional world.

"Where are you? Why aren't you home yet?" my husband asks as I call him from the teachers' lounge.

It's 9:00 p.m. in the days just before the dawn of universal cell phone towers and ample service. I'd eaten nothing but a few snacks and bits of candy to stave off low blood sugar. With so much to pull together for the coming weeks, there is no time for a dinner break.

"I'm stopping soon," I say, knowing it is not quite the truth. "My neck and back are hurting, but I'm still working on report cards for tomorrow's conferences. That's all that's left."

"Come home. Now. You've done enough for today." My guardian angel's insistence promises a compromise between my impossible reach for perfection versus reality. I am momentarily lured by his dear words and vision that would let me tag the finish line and allow me rest, if just for tonight.

"Almost done," I reiterate. "But I'm calling to tell you that my blood sugar won't come down. It crashed two hours ago, so I ate some candy. Thirty minutes ago, my meter said 475. My eyes are throbbing. Everything is throbbing. I'm aching and itchy. I even punched in an extra-large insulin bolus, but it's not working."

"Sweetie, come home." Again, the siren sings.

"It's so dark outside. Pitch black."

My voice breaks involuntarily and against my better judgment. My abilities are slipping away. I can feel it.

I confess, "I'm nervous about walking to my car alone at this time of night."

My school is located near The University of New Mexico in a relatively safe neighborhood adjacent to a park. That park, beautiful by day, has a reputation. Locals call it "Pervert Park," noting that you never know who might emerge from its bowels at night. In my aching, exhausted state, egged on by soaring glucose levels, my reasoning skills scatter. Urban myth meets emotional overload, causing panic and the inability to make an independent, rational decision despite that heady Fulbright award hanging over my head. Befuddled, I hear myself whining, even though I want to choke the woman I've become. Who invited her to the party—this whimpering, pitiful mess? I don't like her at all.

"Driving down right now to meet you," my knight in shining armor says.

I wonder if he senses my paralysis or hears my fear of what isn't working to keep my diabetes at bay.

"We'll change your pump as soon as we get home, okay, hon?"

I don't know what I've ever done, on this precious earth, to earn such a gracious and generous partner, but I crumble and give in to a tear running down my face.

"All right?" he says.

"Yes," I whisper. "Thank you."

Humbled and silenced, both by his act and my inability to multitask or think, I stack the remaining paperwork. Some of it will have to be tackled during tomorrow morning's recess and by adding a fun art-journal activity designed to keep my kiddos quiet and creatively engaged, thus buying me more prep time before the next set of parents arrive for their meeting.

At work the next day, I am tired but focused. Deadlines have a way of commandeering that high level of attention. The countdown toward needed preparation wraps me in its net, and I am aware of little else. As the school day ends, the same pattern of a rebounding glucose level appears: climbing blood sugars unresponsive to the extra boluses I administer every two hours. What is going on?

I push through more grading and summary reports for my last set of conferences. Just two more days to get through, and I'll be on a plane to San Francisco and overseas. I can almost touch the image in my mind, it is so close. But sharp pains begin to intrude. My eyes ache—seemingly swimming in sugar water and blurring my vision. The pit of my stomach rebels like the onslaught of a virulent flu strain. My upper body is consumed with maddening itching that can't be relieved. I pull out my meter: 526. Seemingly impossible as I haven't eaten much all day.

Struggling to breathe, I walk into the teachers' lounge and, in a nod to accepting help, call my nearby endocrinologist's office.

"Mary, can I come over again?" I ask, fighting rapid breaths. "I need someone to help me replace the infusion set for my pump. I don't have any supplies with me at work and I can hardly think, my blood sugar is so high."

"What are you running, sweetie?"

"Over 500. Second day in a row," I report.

"Get over here and we'll see what we need to do."

I dump paperwork into my schoolbag and drag myself to my car and over to the Diabetes Clinic at Lovelace Hospital. Over two hours later, a nurse helps me off the exam table where I've slept in near-coma oblivion. She disconnects the intravenous feed of insulin and electrolytes. My ketones are sky high and a noteworthy shade of deep purple—something I haven't experienced since early college days.

"You should feel better soon," she says. "Go home and get some sleep."

The next day, I feel shaky but hopeful the tide has turned.

Two days later, stress hormones sideline me again. I drive the few miles, once more, to the clinic where a friendly nurse willingly connects me to another insulin drip. It's not my favorite experience, but there's really no other choice.

Two or three emergencies in one week is a lot for anyone who tries their hardest not to let diabetes overrule their lives. There are a mere four days until my awaited flyaway; a deadline practically too close for comfort. Insulin resistance is the apparent culprit; lack of sleep and too much stress hormone, the primary contributing factors. And none of my equipment or my years of knowledge seem to give me sufficient warning or data to know what to do considering the circumstances I face.

Now, I can't help but wonder how having a trained DAD, markedly one who alerts to high glucose levels, might have nipped this pattern. My problem with insulin resistance, which lasted well into my Fulbright trip to Japan, might never have been. A dog like Abbey could have kept me better tuned to those rising sugars. DADs are able to detect real-time sugar levels twenty minutes prior to data provided by home glucose meters. This makes a well-trained DAD a useful and typically dependable tool in one's diabetes toolkit!

More recently, I have found that a CGM teamed with consistent home glucose checks and an insulin pump are all invaluable tools. But there are still problems inherent in overreliance on this technology that make having a trained DAD an asset. Like me, my friends with T1 note that they struggle with false data sometimes supplied by these sensors and monitors. Another challenge is present in not always hearing the system alarms designed to alert wearers to very low or high glucose levels—mainly during sleep. My own experience demonstrates how quickly I have learned to tune out such intrusive noises until the very nature of an audible alert becomes nearly invisible. Or the times when my CGM-insulin pump combination won't stop screeching low blood sugar alerts—many of them unfounded—on a low threshold suspend program.

In an attempt to address these issues and back up my own safety net for nighttime lows, I set up a second doggie doorbell system with the PebbleSmart Doggie Doorbell and place the ringer on the headboard of my bed. Then I proceed to work with Abbey to remind her of my expectations for getting needed alerts.

One summer night, we finally settle in together on an abundant number of pillows topping clean-scented sheets. Abbey curls closely by my side, Tess lies on a bedside chair, and Zoe snuggles by Bob's feet. Hours of earlier garden work have taken their toll as we all fall asleep under the caress of a soft fan.

Beep, beep, beep.

"What?! Not again!"

It's after 1:00 a.m.

First, I do what any practical, too-busy-to-take-time-to-figure-out-the-meaning-of-this-intrusive-situation person might do: I swear. Then I reluctantly drag myself from bed and move online in a desperate search for what the alarm means and how to circumvent the annoying sound coming from my new pump. There are no easy answers here—even in a topic search. I grab my guide book and manhandle it, stumbling through the index and contents to secure relief. There are no definitive answers at my beck and call here either. Finally, at 2 a.m., I call the help desk but get no answer.

I am so frustrated that my most untold thoughts are being muttered aloud. And these would definitely scare a number of people who claim to know me.

At 4 a.m., I call again. Bingo! After winding my way through the automated system and waiting for what seems like forever, a patient care representative answers.

"This is John. How can I help you?"

My heart is hammering with competing beats of hope and irritation.

"My meter is telling me I'm above 75. I've had recent readings of 80, 88, 92 and 75. I'm using your new CGM system, and it won't stop screaming at me about my blood sugar being below 60. What. Is. Going. On?" I try leveling my voice so that I don't lose my cool.

"Even my dog isn't alerting me to low blood sugar, and she is almost always right." I can't help adding this comment.

A few moves later, the voice at the other end helps me reset some programs to reduce the excessive alerts, although I am no further along in understanding what triggered the false CGM readings. I end our phone connection, craving some much-needed sleep.

Yet I can't stop feeling that there's more to this story. Something doesn't quite fit into my hoped-for alliance with my new pump and its integrated CGM. What is it that's nagging at me?

It hits like a jolt from the technology quagmire. While I know there's a lot to learn about this new set-up, it was my trained girl Abbey who stood next to me, watching and indicating there was no real emergency. This time around, my DAD outsmarted my technology.

How fortunate that she was with me. Her input in this most recent challenge seems to have made a difference between other choices I might have made and actions I might have taken—some of them being even downright dangerous. This realization helps me understand how important it is to pull information from many tools designed to inform me about my health. Today, while I might chalk up my good fortune to serendipity, my thoughts linger on what my dog was telling me then; that everything is all right. How many other times has Abbey let me know that I can trust her trained input when the technology, for one reason or another, has provided faulty data or stopped working? She has been proving her worth by coming through for me more times, of late, than I can count.

With all these questions colliding, a spark of newfound energy propels me to lump all my health management tools together. What do I use most and less often to help manage my diabetes? What's invaluable in my day-to-day life? I defer sleep, instead choosing to list what I use on the computer—a technology I appreciate in its straightforward ability to keep me from losing my hand-written lists that manage to float all over my home.

My thinking is hampered by the recent incident, and I start my list ever so slowly:

T1 management tools & technology I use!

- Glucose readings on blood sugar meter ~5-8x/day
- CGM readings + data (as I begin to use them. Starting to wear a CGM sensor 1-3 weeks/month. Analyze patterns in the data.)
- Ketone check (occasional)
- 4+ times/year LAB test results

My thoughts are sluggish, and no wonder—the hour! But once engaged, my brain jumpstarts and the list grows:

PHYSICAL SYMPTOMS—

LOWS: shaking/trembling, headaches, feelings of desperation to stop that shakiness

HIGHS: creeping sensation of deep, internal itching on my back, shoulders, chest, skin. Eyes hurting. Vision blurred.

INSULIN PUMP—internal programs with data-keeping ability (every day 24/7!)

HA1C (Use to measure average of 3 months' sugar levels. Helps me look at insulin amounts programmed into my pump when I find significant patterns of lows and highs)

MEDICAL TEAM—Appointments/questions/problem-solving: with my endocrinologist, Endo PA, Primary Care doc, podiatrist, pump and CGM reps

TIME IN RANGE—(starting to analyze)

DIABETES GROUPS—Joslin Clinic Medalist group & local T1 group

T1 INFO—Diabetes conferences, books, magazine articles

THE DOG

What? How did that last thought sneak through? I take a long look: "The Dog?" Yes, the evidence sits in front of me on an LED-lit screen and with that very dog by my side.

I invariably meet people who hint or boast that of all the tools available to support living with diabetes, a DOG must be the least trustworthy. Something on which you can't count; a variable on which you shouldn't count. I see the skepticism in their body language, most of all when they advocate for the scientific accuracy or relative infallibility of technology. "Compared to a dog," they say.

But, in fact, I am finding that a well-trained DAD like mine demonstrates a keen, consistent ability to detect different and more real-time glucose levels than possible with a blood sugar meter. Most important, I've documented Abbey's responses to low glucose levels to be a vital tool to *include* in a diabetes toolkit—realizing that nothing we use is one hundred percent accurate all of the time. My DAD has saved me countless times already. Her alerts are typically valid. Abbey's ability to detect out-of-range glucose levels are needed—particularly when my insulin or batteries or infusion set or CGM go haywire. Because there are so many worries about equipment malfunction when living diabetes, my dog is a welcome support.

I plan to double down on increasing Abbey's ability to give me nighttime alerts—particularly when the diabetes technology, on which I rely, goes wrong. Getting a nighttime alert is essential, so it doesn't matter what its source. It might come from a DAD, parent, significant other, CGM linked to a watch alarm, or another means. It remains a cornerstone to keeping most people with diabetes healthy and moving forward.

In our first year of DAD training, though I am still fighting my hound's deepest pack-nesting instincts when she is tucked under blankets dreaming the golden dream of hounds chasing bunnies across endless fields, she delivers an overall alert rate of close to 80% over a 24-

hour period, and an 85-90% accuracy rate during her waking hours. My intent is to train harder to generalize Abbey's reliability so that she grows even more dependable over time. With more work and a few creative twists on nighttime alert training, this goal can be achieved.

It's a touch of magic: this quixotic mix of tapping into canine ability, behavior training methods, and strengthening the ties between dogs and humans. The science behind the shaping of a DAD is unfolding as a strong component to all the other informative tools used to support living well with this disease.

I, for one, love counting on Abbey's alerts. I laugh with delight when her amazing ability to scent shows up the most sophisticated technology. While I am thankful for all the technology and scientific knowledge available to me and believe in accessing and using them fully, the one tool that's most untapped is the one I've come to count on—a DAD. I've found no other single tool that can do so much 24/7 with such a subtle, loving and skilled presence: alerting to out-of-range glucose levels in real time, shaping her human handler into an active team leader committed to taking control of diabetes, alleviating the darkest days of loneliness and isolation that come with challenges, and sculpting a magical meeting of hearts and minds through building an empowering life-changing team. Including a DAD as a management tool brings unbridled joy; a significant gain in quality of life issues to live my very best life. Happiness-bound, that's what I seek and swear by. Sometimes, the dog really is smarter.

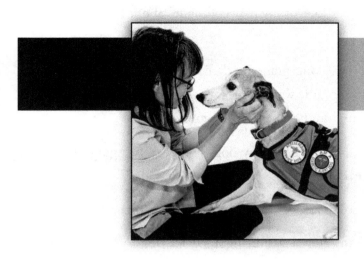

Chapter 19

A DAD In The Workplace?

I start a new school year at Georgia O'Keeffe Elementary in the Northeast Heights—thrilled to be teaching in a unique program with a stellar group of colleagues led by an accomplished principal and eager-to-learn students. But even this positive scenario doesn't fill the gap from missing my girl Abbey, made more poignant a loss by seeing my new community of parents, students and staff welcome a rotation of lovable, tail-wagging therapy dogs. The school's and families' endorsement embraces a belief that therapy dogs are capable of motivating student learning, bridging children's emotions and shaping a stronger, more caring and child-centric community. One small measure of this consensus is evidenced by the stashes of doggie treats kept in many classrooms. Another is the visiting therapy dog schedule posted on classroom doors and printed in the school's online newsletter. It is an unanticipated thrill to find myself in such a place, and it propels me to ask a few questions of my new colleagues about bringing a service dog to school.

"Ann," I ask a second grade teacher two rooms from my own, "is Rio trained in any specific way or through a certified program? And how often do you bring him here to be with your students?"

She answers, "Rio is a therapy dog. I've been bringing him to my class for three years now. He's so good with the kids."

I take a chance to ask her my simmering question.

"I'm wondering how I can bring a service dog to school with me. Do you know anything about who I should check with or what I need to do? I thought you might be able to give me more information since you have permission to bring your own dog here."

"Nope." She shrugs. "Sorry. I only know about therapy dogs. Good luck, though," she warmly replies.

On Friday, I lightly tap on Ann's classroom door during my afternoon recess, which is scheduled at an earlier time than the primary grades' slot. She motions for me to enter as she moves around the room, encouraging her students to finish their literature dioramas and begin clean-up before lining up for recess. Rio lays on the classroom carpet next to a young girl reading him a story. His head is tilted in terrier-style that seemingly says "you are my one and only." My heart expands seeing her trying to explain an illustration as she huddles, nose-to-nose, to talk with her canine partner. A short ten minutes later, I thank Ann and let her know I have to get back to my room as my own students are returning to class.

"I'll have Rio here next week. Come by again on Wednesday if you can," she says.

"How often is he here?" I ask.

"Twice a week."

"He stays all day? What do you do if he has to go potty?"

"I just take him out at recess. It's never a problem. See you on Wednesday or Friday?"

I nod and make a mental note to enter the visit into my busy schedule.

The next two months pass in a blur of holding parent meetings, planning curricula and teaching. Still, my question and intense desire infiltrate my days. At home, I pepper Bob with nonstop scenarios and questions. He knows less than my colleague but believes that I should do what is right for me. And somehow, I know this, too. I bait myself with wondering how much longer I can truly wait before moving ahead with the next step.

I stop into the office before Thanksgiving to ask our school secretary Mrs. Romero about setting up an appointment with the principal, only to discover that she is on medical leave through winter vacation. I am more than a little disappointed. That evening, I email her about Abbey and my wish to bring my DAD to school with me.

As an educator well-versed on Section 504 plans and with a general knowledge of the Americans with Disabilities Act, I feel somewhat secure about my rights. I know what most people know about protection from discrimination and maybe a bit more; that these federal laws clearly support me bringing Abbey to work. Still, my request could be "a first" at my school. This makes it more difficult to determine what my course of action should be. What channels within the school system are in place to help me? What steps are required? The fact is that I don't really know the specifics—even after decades spent as a general and special education teacher and district-level trainer. I have my contacts and guesses, but I'd never yet personally called on these laws in my entire Albuquerque Public Schools career. I never thought I'd need them.

For years, I determined not to make waves in the workplace with any personal requests related to my diabetes; to keep my status as a model employee and an ultimate professional. Who was I fooling? Now, with a clearer understanding of my health needs, I realize the importance of putting supports in place irrespective of my reputation as a teacher. Finally, having lived through trial and error, I am ready to state what I need and bank on these laws as necessary.

Despite my private bravado, the email I send my principal is one that takes a more polite tone. One with which I am comfortable. It seemingly allows me to go through the back door to bring my DAD to my professional workplace. Sending a digital communication gives my principal a chance to share facts with other district staff. It provides her time to look into any work-related issues and check with district lawyers on how to best respond. I know that this is a better way; a dose of honey to sweeten the relationship, interactions and decisions. I realize, too, that it's not the only route open to me.

While a decision brews, I decide to be proactive and draft a letter to my students' parents. At the earliest, a positive response to my inquiry might allow me to bring my girl in mid-January. Too soon, I reason; a better starting date is February because it will give more time for holding class discussions, setting rules and norms and determining which of my students are committed to working with Abbey as my initial helpers for on-site training. Grappling with my self-imposed delay in introducing Abbey to school, I draft my letter and hold it in reserve to share with my principal for her feedback once a district decision is made. I read the letter over and over in the weeks before returning to school—tweaking a sentence here and there, adding room for questions and comments and embellishing it with Abbey's photo.

Dear Parents,

I plan to bring a special dog named Abbey into class on 1-2 teaching days each week beginning February 2015. Abbey, a 2 ½ year old whippet, is intelligent, loving and sociable. Having her in class would provide much insight for our children into the exceptional capabilities of service dogs, even teaching some dog-training and animal care skills to those most interested in these types of canines. A number of (our school's) teachers bring therapy dogs into the school and classrooms—with very beneficial learning impact on our students!

The behavioral standards for training a service dog are very high. Abbey has received specialized training as a Diabetes Alert Dog (or DAD) for just under a year, to date, and she consistently receives ongoing reinforcement training. Further, she is continuously guided to comply with nationally recognized public behaviors that include these types of commands: sit, wait, stay, drop, down, no touch/leave it. Best behaviors are important for all canines, and they are a basic expectation for service dogs of all types.

Your children and I have discussed the possibility of Abbey attending class, as well as how to support anyone who experiences allergies to dogs. For your information, Abbey's coat is very short-haired, so she only sheds a small amount. If your child has allergies, we can have your child sit further from the dog, and wash his/her hands after touching her, if this would be helpful. Please contact me, via the note below, email, or stopping by the classroom, if you have any concerns about your child, and I will support whatever steps are needed to ensure your child's health.

Please return the form, below, with your signature giving permission for your child to be in contact (or limited contact) with Abbey. Thank you.

Sincerely,

Kathy Richter-Sand, Ed.D (and Abbey)

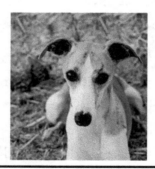

I attach a second section for parents and students to fill out and return. Necessary? Not really. But it's designed with a gentle approach toward bringing a DAD into the classroom and opening the door to positive home-school communication. I want to give families a chance to address parental concerns, list questions and share specific requests for their children when Abbey comes into class.

Abbey is a Service Dog working with her trainer and human partner Katherine Richter-Sand, a teacher at GOK Elementary. Abbey is a 2½ year old short-coated whippet who is up-to-date on all shots. She is professionally trained according to National Public Access Behaviors and meets all requirements of a Service Dog as defined by Federal Law.

If you AGREE that your child may be in the classroom with this dog, please sign and return this slip to school. If your child has any specific needs in terms of allergies or another issue, please note this information, below.

—— —— —— —— —— ——

My child has my permission to be in class with

Abbey, a Service Dog, for the remainder of the school year.

I have the following questions/concerns:

—— —— —— —— —— ——

When there is nothing more to change or add, I reluctantly put everything aside. Finally, vacation ends and I head back to work, leaving Abbey at home. I find myself inundated with the new year's schoolwide student achievement testing, writing IEP updates, scheduling spring family transition meetings for my graduating fifth graders heading to our middle schools and finalizing my own professional portfolio for the yearly assessment of my teaching goals. Faced with this onslaught of tasks, all thoughts or hopes I have of hearing anything about bringing

Abbey to school are buried under deep layers of paperwork and the rush of a new semester. Nearly forgotten for now, I have little choice but to put my deepest wish on hold.

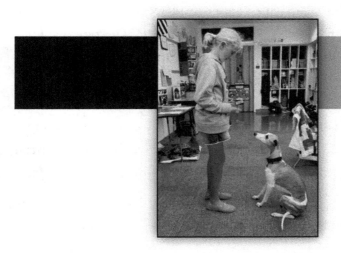

Chapter 20

Team Abbey Moves Forward

Just seven days into the new year, the email I have long awaited, but have been too preoccupied to address, arrives with a "ping" in my mailbox. Busy working with various student science groups, there is no time to open and view any incoming mail until dismissal time, but I somehow know that an official response, sent through my principal, awaits. Every fiber and hair seem to quiver on my body; that email determines my future with my treasured girl Abbey—at least in a professional context. Dramatic? Yes. But it feels that intense—our deep bond so profoundly strengthened by the lifesaving work she's been trained to do. This is something I've wanted and needed—to have my dog with me—for the longest time.

Prior to returning to school in January, there had been an ample interval for deliberation about taking this possible new path. Moving forward and bringing Abbey as my DAD into my much-coveted

149

professional realm—one in which I am considered a master teacher, like many others in my new community—isn't a choice I question. I am not overly worried about having to cope with intrusive personal questions about my dog's role as a service dog, as my colleagues and this community tend to respect such boundaries. Some of my concerns have been eased by our participation and enthusiastic reception at a number of New Mexico community health fairs, endorsed by the American Diabetes Association, helping me grapple with questions people ask about Diabetic Alert Dogs.

What still troubles me is my inability to answer, for myself, what seems the biggest and most personal query of all; one that someone in my workplace may very well ask: What are the reasons why someone who has lived reasonably well without a DAD suddenly needs to bring along a service dog to her professional workplace? It's a challenging question; one I find a bit too intrusive to tackle with a simple reply to school administrators who don't know me.

All things in good time, I remind myself. My eager-to-learn students clamor for attention and bring my focus back to the here and now.

"Hurry up, my chickadees. It's time to clean up!"

Minutes later, I hear the dismissal bell chime three times, and then I wave my angels out the door.

"Bye, Dr. R-S!" they sing in near-unison. Hands wave and feet move forward, tripping one kiddo into the next like an uneven domino stack. They giggle in delight at the tumultuous departure routine.

"See you tomorrow," I call back.

Inevitably there is a path of forgotten and unseen items strewn in their exuberant wake: erasers, pencils and pens, rulers, school notes meant for parents, flash drives, partially eaten snacks tumbled out of open student lockers. Just like Hansel and Gretel's path, I note to myself. It's funny how some things never change.

"Now I can finally sit down and read through my emails," I say aloud to no one in particular after swooping to straighten up the classroom and posting tomorrow's schedule on the whiteboard. The day, like every other day of engaged instruction, has tapped me dry. Teaching is like staging a play for multiple audiences, one performance after another. I love the interactions with students and colleagues, as well as the detailed work required to plan meaningful new learning experiences. Today, though, I am depleted. Abbey is not with me, and all I really want is to head home where she and her two packmates await my return.

The computer screen resets as I scan the day's list of new communications. There it is. Just one that calls me to open it; the rest can wait.

In a seemingly out-of-body experience, my eyes record the image of a simple touch—my finger pressing on the keyboard and opening my principal's note four hours after its arrival. I read silently, eagerly, perched on the edge of my chair.

I hope you enjoyed your winter vacation. I am recuperating well from my surgery and expect to be back at school soon.

In response to your email request about having your service dog accompany you to school, you may proceed at any time. We are happy to have her join our community.

I look forward to seeing you with Abbey soon. In the meantime, please let me know if you have any questions or issues that arise.

My state of exhaustion dissipates even before my brain reads the last lines. I sit rigidly upright in a state of disbelief and anticipation; hyper-focused on the words in front of me.

Read it again just to be sure. I do so with adrenaline pumping.

Okay, then, you're not crazy. Time to celebrate.

Recalling that I'd earlier closed my classroom door after my students' exit, I allow myself a moment of sheer joy; a triumphant screech that otherwise might have resounded down the hallway and caused nearby teachers to investigate. But my joyous hurrah is safely contained.

I dial my husband's cell.

"The person you are trying to reach is unavailable. Please leave a message at the beep."

Dang it; he must be in a meeting.

"Bob," I record, "you need . . . just call me right away when you finish your meetings and I have amazing news and the best opportunity just happened."

How he'd find a way to decipher the voicemail was beyond me, as my breathless state makes my words trip over each other. Intent on rushing home, I throw a few stacks of papers in need of grading into my ginormous teaching bag—despite knowing they won't be touched tonight.

I drive homeward in a dreamlike state filled with imaginings of bringing Abbey with me and my students' interaction with her. I know the details are crucial; deciding on the when, where and how cannot be underestimated. The key to success, as many before me have said, is in the planning.

I pull into the driveway just as Bob calls.

"So?" he says. I can tell he already knows by the smile I hear and sense on his face. He doesn't have to say much else.

"Fantastic news, I'll bet," he teases. "I'm already on my way. Let's celebrate with dinner out tonight."

"Sweetie, I'm too tired. Would you pick up some dinner and bring it home?"

"That will work," my faithful supporter agrees. "See you soon."

I step inside and head right to the dog kennel to give the dogs free reign. They bark and trot with complete abandon, stopping in short bursts for hugs and toys to be tossed for the chase.

"C'mon, girls, let's go get some supper."

Abbey moves in closest to me, claiming her alpha position. I stop to hold her face and tell her the good news. All I care about is that she feels the depth of love I bear for her, and she seems to acknowledge it with an extra glow in her eyes that gaze deep into my psyche. I can't help but stop for a moment, moved by this miraculous connection, before we all bounce toward the kitchen.

Tonight, I will plan the first day Abbey will accompany me to school as well as the needed preparations for my students and their parents. How many days I'll bring Abbey remains to be seen, But working just a few days per week, my responsibilities each week are immense. Those at-work hours include seeing parents for conferences and IEP meetings, planning with colleagues, implementing gifted curricular instruction and organizing special education-related paperwork. I realize that the demands of my job may only allow me to bring Abbey one day each week without major distraction from my professional duties.

Still, it's a start. Another world has opened; one filled with fascinating possibilities. I can't wait to see how our hard work pays off. Surely, Team Abbey will transform my own experience and the lives of those around me in ways I have not yet fathomed.

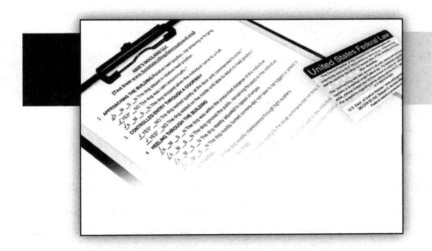

Chapter 21

The Assistance Dog Public Access Behavior Test

May 23 looms large, double-boxed on my calendar in yellow and red marker, as the last time I'd have to prove to Arie that Team Abbey has worked diligently enough to pass the Assistance Dog Public Access Test. Six days remain for practicing every command, making certain it's all routine, well understood and executed without any hesitation on either my part or Abbey's.

The truth is hard to swallow; that this is our second formal testing, so I wonder if Arie has any specific concerns. I don't think so, but it's possible. Months ago, our first assessment seemed to prove Abbey's worthiness for being out in public. She had performed exceptionally well on all the required behaviors. But the testing needed more distractions than we could find—mostly in the form of noisy children and interactions with strangers at the typically busy Coronado Mall.

Lacking these chaotic factors, we'd arranged for an additional assessment. If we do well this time around, Arie will sign us off for meeting the standards for all the behaviors expected of any service dog out in public places. I will then have the right to take Abbey into most places, backed by federal law. But even more important is having deep confidence in my dog and her skills; to me, that is worth more than anything.

Knowing the stakes gives me a strong sense of responsibility to continue working with Abbey and mastering all of these standards. Though the training is fun, it's a serious business; service dogs are not granted much leeway for any troublesome conduct once trained to the highest level. I understand that every behavior from my dog should be dependable. I know only too well that no annoying habits or socially undesirable behaviors are tolerated without consequences or even disqualification as a service dog. As in, there will be no excuses allowed if Abbey "happens" to put her paws onto a food service counter at the coincident time she smells something familiar or enticing. Yes, I plead guilty to sharing kernels of popcorn and occasionally mixing tidbits of safe-to-eat human foods into her dry kibble. What I know and fear, despite my disbelief when watching begging-for-food scenes from any of my dogs, is that they never forget a smell or taste to which they have been introduced. This temptation with familiar smells and tastes worries me, and I can't help but wonder if handler error, in the end, will betray me.

I've awakened most days and this looming week, in particular, hoping I've taught my dog well enough over the last year to avoid any glitches in her execution of public access behavior expectations. And although alerting to low blood sugars and other specific DAD training behaviors are not part of the criterion for the Public Access Behavior

Test, it all has to be wrapped into our training with the same high expectations and standards. Nothing I can think of has been left for granted or untrained—except for future DAD training tasks too complex to tackle at this time. It's a lot to take in, but after so much coaching and instruction, I imagine we'll make the grade. But then, I'm not the examiner assessing whether Abbey truly meets these generally agreed-upon national standards. My heart flutters a bit at this thought.

I rise on testing day to the typical skies for which New Mexico is renown: cloudless, piercing blue and promising the burgeoning warmth of spring bursting into early fragrant bloom. Abbey's service vest, plush mat, drinking water and cup, the ever-present poop bags, and a treat pouch sit on the kitchen counter. In usual fashion, I sing out loud to all three girls, "You are my sunshine, my only sunshine, you make me happy when skies are grey, you'll never know, dears, how much I love you, I am blessed by your love each day."

I laugh at my cheesy rendition; notes of sheer happiness meant to power me through the coming challenge and a reminder of how this love and devotion have lightened my diabetes-related worries in every way. They connect us, and that means everything. They are often the difference between moving forward or giving in to a very dramatic pity party. But where would I be then?

"Let's get breakfast, girls," I say after throwing on a pair of jeans and watching the dogs bask in my attention.

I check Abbey, knowing she shouldn't eat much because a large meal will make her sleepy and inattentive. I measure a tiny amount of kibble into her bowl and stand there on high alert, not putting it past her to intimidate her sisters from their rightful bowls or to inhale their kibble when they become distracted. Alphas just know how to lay claim to the food lottery, winning the ultimate survival prize in the animal kingdom. But it isn't going to happen today, of all days, on my watch.

I leash Abbey for a quick walk around the block. Her sisters Tess and Zoe stare with mournful, accusatory eyes when no additional leashes are pulled.

"C'mon, Abs, let's head out for a practice run."

She bolts in delight from the kitchen into the doorway to the garage. I block the other two from moving forward.

"Sorry, girls, just Abbey this morning." My back remains to them since my sense of guilt is weighty at leaving them behind, and I can't look into their eyes without caving.

"Okay, Abs, let's review some of these things." I carry the folded pages of our upcoming test in my hand as we set out.

"Sit," I tell her while watching for a quick response. Then, "Down."

This command is not easily executed by sighthounds on hard surfaces, but we've trained this one over and over, so I expect and get her willing compliance.

"Good girl!" I sing her praises for reinforcement. Not that she needs this, but it makes me feel good. We relax and take in the humming sounds of yard work welcoming the day before heading home.

Time slows to a crawl. Each fifteen minutes seems like an hour as I wait for the oven timer to sound; a reminder of when to hustle out to meet Arie at Costco—her choice of location based on its popularity and hubbub, including having close turns around laden displays and the lure of readily accessible, wafting food samples. This is a place filled with potential traps—exactly what makes it as perfect a testing site as can be conjured.

Bzzz. Bzzz. Bzzz.

The sound unnerves me. Lost in emails and writing, I'd finally let go of my spiraling anticipation and watching the timer tick down. "Abbey?" I call. But she is nowhere in sight. I find her outside with Tess, both of them sitting silent and sphinxlike, just as eons of ancient sighthounds have done before them, in a sunny spot within the adobe-walled courtyard.

"Hey, girls," I counter. "Let's come inside now and cool down."

Minutes later, I strap Abbey into her service vest and collar. The trusty treat pouch is clipped onto my waistband. I gather my carry bag of dog supplies and grab for the matching service dog mat made by Francie. Juggling skills, I note, would be a definite asset. They're on my wish list but it's much too late to count on them now.

Abbey and I move out of the house and into the car. Just minutes later, we park in Costco's lot and I call Arie to let her know we've arrived. She has asked me to wait for her arrival so she can check our unloading procedure—just one of the behaviors for keeping a service dog safely under control (this one, a controlled exit out of a vehicle, which must be observed).

"All right, Abs, I see her," I say out loud.

Arie waves and signals that it's fine to get out of the car.

Focus and everything will work out perfectly.

I smile at her, opening my door and giving her a quick hug.

"Ready?" she asks.

"Absolutely," I reply, handing her a new copy of the Assistance Dog Public Access Test she asked me to bring. In all honesty, I am sure she has an ulterior motive; something akin to having me review all of the expectations since she could have easily accessed this information herself. A smart move, I think.

"Then let's do it!" she says brightly, as if ringing a starting bell.

I move to the passenger door, open it and gesture a "wait" command for Abbey while I lean down to feel the temperature of the asphalt. I know well, by this point in our training, that if it's too hot, a service dog must be carried, whenever possible, to a nearby cooler surface.

"Feels fine," I say, totally focused on my dog. I check all around me for any potentially dangerous conditions or distractions. Clear. Then I attach her lead, release her car harness and gather her things.

"Abbey, bingo. Jump."

With that, my girl jumps down from her seat and quietly waits for me to lock the car before we head calmly toward the front of the store. It is already filled with customers.

"Kat, you'll just kind of walk with Abbey and stay in front of me or nearby when you get inside. That way, I can watch you and work through the list. How's that sound?"

I nod, keeping my dog in a heel position without pulling too tightly on her lead. It is forbidden for an Assistance Dog to forge ahead or lag behind, and no fear can be exhibited—not at cars, surrounding noises or people coming and going.

I grab a shopping cart from the queue and watch Abbey move like a natural to the front left side. At the store's entrance, despite the greeter welcoming us, I stop; another requirement. "The dog must not pull or strain against the lead or try to push its way past the individual but must wait patiently while entry is completed." She does the right thing. Again, negotiating safe entry is the goal. From the corner of my eye, I see Arie writing something, but in any case, I'm pleased. We walk into the warehouse.

Business is booming but Abbey stays focused on my pace. This is precisely what she needs to do . . . turn corners carefully, follow my speed and move through busy areas without her attention straying far from me. Arie repositions us here and there with, "Let's turn right. Stop. Okay, move forward and turn the next corner." These functions are required—Command #4, called "Heeling through the building."

We stop to pick up a few items, and then Arie says, "She's doing great. Now let's do a six-foot recall on lead."

I move to a more open aisle and signal Abbey to sit. Then I step away, more than the required six feet from her, pretend-shopping for various items on the shelves. Abbey watches but doesn't seem worried. I turn to my trainer for her cue.

"Now, call her to you."

"Abbey, come." She travels a straight line and sits like a beautiful statue in front of me.

Oh, happy day. My internal smile feels like it's a mile wide.

"What a good little doggie you are, Ms. Abster," Arie praises as she motions us forward again.

When we are walking again at a fast pace, Arie says abruptly, "Ask her to sit."

I do, and Arie immediately asks, "Are you ready?" as she picks up a heavy packet of notepads. I know what's coming but before I can nod "yes," she drops it behind us. It slams onto the floor with a loud bang. Abbey glances in her direction but her demeanor stays calm and collected. No aggression. No shaking or fear. Not even any tangible "startle reaction."

That's my girl.

"I'm really impressed," Arie says. "I can tell she's been out a lot with you. A lot. Just amazing."

I smile. If Abbey could simply smile, I'm certain she would right now. Maybe she is beaming in her own way hearing Arie's comments. It's a funny thought; one that makes me intently study her face.

"Now we're going to go to the food court and I'll check her sits, stays and downs. How's a juicy slice of pizza sound?" she asks.

I answer silently. *Could be Purgatory.* Aloud, I say, "Okay."

My voice is overly cheerful and high-pitched in an attempt to convince myself, and my dog, that anything is possible. I just hope we err on the side of success.

On our way to the front of the store, I stop and pay for the few items picked up during this trip. Proper check-out protocol is essential here, too. I place my dog in a sit-stay command slightly in front of me as I pull out a bank card. The cashier is trying her hardest not to lean over and coo to Abbey—seeing that we are working hard to do everything according to procedure. Arie is off to the side, watching us with a quirky half-smile on her face as she's prone to do. It's hard to interpret any judgments she has made, but I know for certain that there is nothing she doesn't see.

Once we exit the checkout line, Arie asks me to find a table and wait. I motion Abbey to come beside me on her padded mat at a table closest to the exiting beeline of customers. Despite the risk of people stopping to pet her and talk with me, it seems easier than wiggling through the maze of close-set tables on the furthest side.

"Abbey, under," I order: a safety measure. She tucks her body partway beneath the table legs. We wait for Arie's return, and she joins us within minutes with a steaming pizza slice—so hot and oversized that cheese is oozing onto the paper plate and over its edges.

My mouth waters. Yes, I am weak. What I'd give to gulp that down under different circumstances. But I know it's not for me, and that issue, in itself, seems cruel. I give up predicting what might happen and let Arie take command—never before having faced such a juicy, palatable test with Abbey.

Arie is beaming with delight; she obviously loves a challenge. I wonder if she thinks my dog will "cave" on these next three "sit commands" and the two required "down commands." I'm not sure, but seeing my own senses ready to cash it in, I have my doubts that Abbey will be a successful holdout.

"I'm going to put this plate next to Abbey, and I want you to tell her to sit. I won't keep it there too long. We aren't trying to be cruel."

Really? I nod but feel my right eyebrow rise in cynical dissent.

If the saying "misery loves company" has any truth to it, I feel momentarily pressured. All I can think to do is succumb and tell Abbey that it's all right: we can fail together through the commission of gluttony. Instead, I somehow find the presence of mind to nod once more to Arie.

She shoves the mouthwatering plate inches from Abbey's feet. Abbey sits there on my command, without so much as a verbal or physical correction, and ignores the lure.

"Aha! That's really good!" Arie notes. She smiles at me, probably because I sense my mouth opening and closing in disbelief.

"All right, walk her around a bit so she's not so stressed. Then I'll have you give her a 'down' and I'll drop a piece of this on the floor near her."

Abbey and I rise together and as we move into the path of customers, we are besieged with requests for petting, her name, and our purpose there today. We take time to allow for these connections—so important for the both public and my dog—and then I walk her around for a minute.

"Okay, girl, let's go back to the table now."

I'm careful not to pull tightly on her lead, but she doesn't seem upset.

"Abbey, down," I tell her. Then I motion to her mat. "Go mat."

She drops on it, groans and tucks her nose into the cushion's padding. Extracurricular activities always stress canines, and I can see that she's tired and ready to go home.

"Uh oh," interrupts Arie. She rips off a huge piece of the pizza and drops it onto the floor. It lands ten inches from Abbey.

What a waste of really good food. I note that my blood sugar must be dropping since I want to eat every morsel of that succulent piece despite it touching the floor.

"Leave it," I command and, to my astonishment, she does. Some nearby customers watch closely. Comments reflect their interest and approval of Abbey's polished manners.

"What a trooper!" Arie sings.

"Amazing," I concur.

"Yep," says our trainer of few words. "Let's go."

I gather Abbey's Service Dog mat, roll her lead into my hand and we walk in perfect unison out the door—pausing, of course, according to trained Assistance Dog protocol on expected exit technique.

After putting Abbey into the car, I let myself take a huge breath. Like my DAD, I'm drained but exhilarated too.

"So, how'd you think we did?" I ask Arie as she finishes scribbling a few things onto the front of the test.

She smiles, a grin so wide that her eyes seem to disappear like smiley face creases into her face, and she hands me the test. She doesn't really have to say anything, I realize, but I glance down at the cover anyway.

"IT'S A PASS!"

"Take it home, look it over and call me if you have any questions or problems with other things you're training. Good job, girl!" She pats Abbey on the shoulder.

A hug and a quick goodbye later, Abbey and I are homeward bound for a celebration. Treats followed by a nap will be a perfect wrap-up for this coveted day.

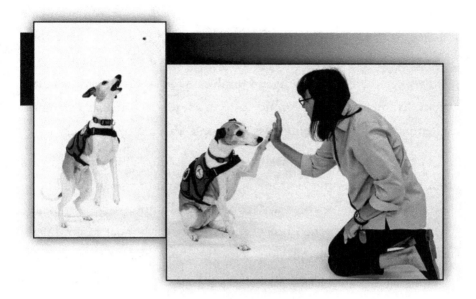

Chapter 22

Adding Gravy: Simple Cues For Alleviating Stress

Being a canine hero or heroine isn't easy. So many people are drawn to dogs, in particular those like Abbey who appear perfectly trained and exude an extraordinary level of understanding and intimacy with their handlers. I've heard people say, "Oh, that dog is working and I know I shouldn't bother them," only to see hands sweep in to stroke her. I remind myself to remain tolerant and calm at these intrusions, seeing how captivated people are; how much they seem to crave this connection and just can't help themselves.

Despite the impositions sometimes presented, people's interest in Abbey is generally welcome. This is because I am pleased that my dog, like all service dogs, is an important delegate for showing the community what she does. She is a well-behaved advocate for anyone touched by diabetes. The proof is found in people who articulate their feelings by telling me that they are deeply moved by our relationship, teamwork, and Abbey's diligent resolve. This is a mighty powerful accomplishment, and I'm proud to have an ally in bringing awareness and empathy to the growing crisis of people affected by diabetes.

There's no doubt that a well-trained service dog of any type garners attention. It strikes me as ironic since a paramount goal for training these dogs is to make them as "invisible" and unobtrusive as possible when carrying out trained tasks in most places. My goal to go quietly on and about my own business? Nearly impossible. Abbey and I are constantly bombarded with questions from people who encounter us in stores or appointments.

The attention bestowed on Abbey—with my watchful permission when she's not in 100% working mode—is what gives me my first inkling that adding to Abbey's skillset beyond public access protocols and DAD training might not be such a bad idea. Several situations form the impetus for this idea: wanting to challenge my dog to learn more; finding ways to keep her from being bored; searching for breaks in her on-the-job routine to alleviate stress; breaking through dubious mindsets held by the most serious doubters.

On a stormy winter's day filled with dark grey skies that smell of incoming snow, I pull out Abbey's most thickly-padded service dog vest for a jaunt to our local Costco.

"Hey, sweet Abs, let's get ready to go pick up a few quick groceries. Come here!"

Abbey trots in her inimitable prance, as only a true diva can, to sit just in front of me. She glances at me, and then past me, trying to ascertain the reason for my call.

"Yes, that's right. We're headed out together. Ready for some fun?" I say while coaxing her to stay still long enough for me to place the heavy vest over her head and secure the mid-body Velcro straps.

She waits and watches, like all good sighthounds, missing nothing. Even when I reach to fill the waist-clipped treat bag with small, dedicated treats only used for DAD training rewards, she quivers in anticipation but continues taking it all in.

I slip on my coat and then attach her black lead to the lined service dog collar handmade by Francie. Abbey's sisters leap around us and thwart an easy exit to the car. Abbey's lead is their clue that we should all be heading out for a walk, and I'm sorry to disappoint them by leaving them behind. My guilt makes me promise them a later jaunt. Then I move to hide treats throughout the den for them to find when I release them from their "stay!" command.

Abbey and I squeeze out the door into the garage as Tess and Zoe scramble frantically to uncover their hidden treasures. Just a few minutes later, the two of us arrive at our destination.

"Let's go inside, girl," I say, releasing Abbey from her position. "Not much time to stroll today. We have to be home soon."

We move into the entrance, my list in hand.

"Ooh, look Mommy, a dog!" I hear a child, strapped into a cart, squeal.

Try to avoid people's eyes. It will go much faster this way.

I'm a woman on a mission—determined to be in and out of the store in twenty minutes. I move forward with my list in hand and desperately trying to avoid eye contact with anyone.

Zipping through the warehouse is an unlikelihood as new products beckon me: 'Buy me now or risk never finding me here again.' The temptation to shop and stroll is overwhelming, and I stop with Abbey while perusing lofty vests and clothing that promise warmth from the coming storm and protection from dark winter days looming ahead.

"Oh my God. Just look at that beautiful dog. I wish I had one like that."

A woman's voice beseeches a nearby friend to take a chance to step into my frame of reference or for me to stop. I don't know which one, but I am firmly trying to ignore her. I smile at her words, hoping that will be enough.

It isn't.

"What does she do?" the nameless, faceless shopper asks.

At that, I glance up.

A middle-aged woman in a wheelchair gazes lovingly at Abbey. Her arms are stiff and misshapen as she reaches toward us. *Multiple sclerosis?* Her legs appear wizened at the years of her condition's toll. My heart cracks at my prior stubborn resolve, now vaporized.

"Hi," I answer softly, moving toward her, Abbey by my side.

"This is Abbey. She's a service dog."

"For you? Or do you train them?" she asks, her wish plastered on her face, eyes as big as saucers.

"Both," I tell her gently. We move closer so she can touch Abbey.

"Ohhh," she murmurs. "I don't live here but I wish you could help me train a dog like her."

Again, she asks, "What can she do?"

I gulp, wondering how much personal information to reveal. I decide to take a chance and unveil the privacy curtain that usually protects me.

"She's trained as a Diabetic Alert Dog," I say. "She can sense and alert to low blood sugar levels."

"That's wonderful," comes the reply.

I breathe a sigh of relief and nod and pivot away from revealing more. "She is learning some tricks too. Would you like to see some?"

The woman gasps. "Really?" Her face is flooded in anticipation.

Again, I nod. "Abbey, turn right. Good girl. Now turn left."

These are basic agility commands and behaviors generally unknown to many people. Abbey and I learned to work agility courses from the time she was a pup. We continue to train together even as our agility classes and DAD training overlap. Abbey's responses to these cues are often viewed as clever tricks when people see how she responds. But their true role, when we travel to unfamiliar environments and interact with strangers, is one that benefits Abbey by reducing her stress level though a simple, quick and fun distraction from the intensity of having to be on constant alert for me. Still, they almost always infuse an enthusiastic response.

The stranger says, "Amazing. I just love her."

I realize, then, that having my DAD perform a simple behavior that is perceived as a "trick" accomplishes something that's not so measurable and has nothing to do with helping me live with my condition: it makes people happy. It draws people in and opens them to learning more about service dogs. A "trick" here and there encourages a desire to find out more about the work and training these dogs receive. The skillset mastered by service dogs gives them a distinct and rightful place in the human world, and any respectful interactions with the public help pave this understanding. When appropriate, these connections can help foster the precious insight that the special bonds between service dogs and their handlers can be nurtured in their own canines. A familiar lump forms in my throat as I think about telling this woman that we have to get going.

"Would you like my email and phone number in case you think of some questions to ask me?" I offer. "Maybe you'll find someone to help you train a dog closer to where you live."

She stares at me with such need that I can only wish this will happen. Loneliness; a desire to love and be loved; a need for trained support that might ease the physical limitations of her visible condition: all these things are expressed in her questions, certainly, but more so in her immediate connection with Abbey who stands quietly by this stranger's side, allowing the woman's gnarled hands to caress her head. For a few minutes, the woman simply beams.

I lean forward, give her an extra-light hug and wish her luck. I know only too well how such a well-trained canine partner can alleviate one's physical burdens and sense of loneliness.

In the time it takes to drive home with Abbey, I take a few minutes to reflect on this unexpected encounter. 'What can she do?' rings in my head. I didn't have to directly answer the question but this is one time that proved it was good to take a chance. The "tricks" routine might be viewed as a pathway to connect with the public but to be tapped only when it's safe to do so.

My classroom—an entirely different setting—further guides my intuition on the role of teaching my dog a few "trick-like" behaviors. Before bringing Abbey into school, I think long and hard about how to present her to my students: What rules do I want them to follow to ensure they treat her with respect? What can I do to involve students in Abbey's training to demonstrate that those whose interactions are marked by a consistently calm, effective and caring demeanor might reap the closest relationships with her? How should our first day together look and sound? And perhaps most important: what do I truly hope to accomplish by sharing Abbey the DAD with my students? The planning is challenging only because of the scope of my dream; a wonderful, life-impacting outcome for my students.

"I'll be bringing Abbey in tomorrow, kiddos," I announce at the close of a busy day.

My students are a group of highly gifted third, fourth, and fifth-graders who pulse with palpable anticipation at finally meeting my dog. They have waited months, like me, for an answer. Still, I realize that the introduction must be limited in length and scope since new scenarios always create stress for dogs.

"When you arrive tomorrow, you will probably want to run in, pet and greet Abbey. How would you feel if she were you?"

"I'd be so scared," says Sasha. "She, I mean I, might pee on the carpet."

The kids fall over in glee at this clever tongue-in-cheek response. I laugh too.

"Yes, we wouldn't want that."

Evan adds, "Maybe we should come in quietly, sort of slink in, and wait for her to come up to us when we're at our desks."

Several children nod their approval.

"Well," I say, "I'm thinking that I want Abbey to get to know each of you and to like you. And that every day she comes to school, our Helper of the Week can pass three or four dog treats out to everyone. Then you can be co-trainers with me, and by giving Abbey a piece of a treat for doing what you ask, she will learn to trust you."

"Yes!" I hear. Several children high-five each other.

"Let's follow this plan for tomorrow and I'll show you how to help Abbey practice a few behaviors. For now, let's pick up scraps off the carpet so that Abbey isn't tempted to eat anything that could hurt her."

They fall onto the carpet, scouring for every dropped paper clip, staple and paper scrap in sight.

"Good job! Abbey and I thank you," I say. "Let's get ready to go now. The bell is about to ring."

As the last student skips out the door, their voices drift back to me.

"All right," they say. "This will be so cool. Our very own class dog."

The next morning when my fifth graders arrive, followed by their younger peers, Abbey is already lying down, napping on her plush service dog mat. She glances up as one child after another takes their place. Up steps our Helper of the Week, eager to assist and expand Abbey's world, thereby transforming the perceptions held by my students and our school community as only children somehow can.

I begin by showing them how to have Abbey "tap" a piece of paper. Then I demonstrate how to ask Abbey to "tap" their palms and thighs, assisted by my volunteer helper. Once we run through more alert behaviors, I move on to a few commands that fall more into the "tricks" category. My students, like most people, are enamored with what Abbey understands.

Are training these few "trick" behaviors inherent to being a great DAD? Of course not, but I realize that Abbey seems to relish learning and performing them. She basks in the "yeses!" that serve as behavior markers. Because boredom is a terrible state for a dog's mind, I want to keep Abbey thinking and working. Learning a few commands outside the role of serving as my DAD gives her purpose by opening up her world to positive social interactions with strangers. Performing these so-called "tricks," when circumstances allow, eases the stress of doing her job. I find that in terms of considering Abbey's personality, all of these elements play into keeping her motivated. Perhaps just as vital, I've found them key to shaping the desired temperament of a DAD and service dog.

It is, admittedly, a controversial path. My efforts to share Abbey and her role with the public violates the key rule about service dogs—to let them focus on their jobs without interruption. It is crucial, in general, that others not impose their desires to meet or touch one of these specifically-trained dogs because the tasks they do are always, in some way, life-saving. Many times their life-saving roles are not so obvious, which makes the canon of "do not touch or interfere with any service dog" so necessarily imperative. Handlers' lives depend on these dogs, and it makes perfect sense that most cannot allow for these interactions, or even consider the luxury of non-essential "trick" behaviors even when meant to relieve a dog's stress or foster "PR." The impact of one's own physical and medical conditions have to drive the ways service dogs are trained and then worked in community settings by their owner-handlers. Ultimately, the golden rule in Service Dogdom necessarily remains focused on supporting every handler's health and quality of life.

In some ways, I am lucky. I think of my DAD as another "tool" in my diabetes management toolkit that provides me with important feedback on the equilibrium of my health. I find her input just as helpful as my reliance on data from my insulin pump and CGM. If I'm able to access the information that these multiple tools provide, I may choose to share this tool—Abbey—with people who express interest. Nothing is a given, but I realize that my stance of allowing interactions, when possible and when not dangerous to my own health, is an exception to what is generally accepted within public domain.

And what about me labeling Abbey—a highly-skilled DAD and occasional trickster—a "tool" in the management of my day-to-day health: is that merely the crux of what a DAD is? I have to wiggle a bit and state that although Abbey *is* this, she is also so much more. She rises above the technology as a living, responsive assistant and team member while providing me with input on my glucose level. She makes the biggest difference through our strong, interactive bond and shared work by helping me forge ahead from merely coping to living with and solving the multitude of emotional and physical challenges I encounter every single day. For me, being accompanied by such a skilled companion with a few behavioral "tricks" up her sleeve—one capable of inspiring awe and helping me laugh in spite of my trials—simply has no equal.

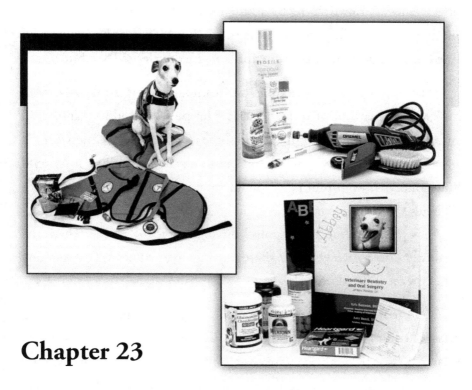

Chapter 23

Be Careful What You Wish For

Most of us struggle to see into the future and understand the unknown, and it has been no different for me as my strong yearning to have a DAD has become a reality. Nothing our trainer Arie shared with me about the depth and 24/7 implications of the relationship between a handler and DAD were fathomable until it evolved into what it is today. I could not have forecasted this future with any accuracy. Now that it's here, I see that the amount of work required to create my "beast of burden," aka Abbey, has been a substantial endeavor.

Training a Diabetic or Diabetes Alert Dog raises many issues and challenges deserving careful reflection. I frequently examine the effectiveness of our training by asking myself these questions: Do I find my trained dog helpful most of the time? (Yes.) Can she be counted on one hundred percent of the time for low glucose alerts? (No, but close.)

The time we've spent shaping our team and Abbey's role as a DAD has elevated her to near-human status. Her position and its standing in my life, and that of my family, has in some inexplicable way transformed her from being a loved animal and pet to a status more like my friend and cohort, now profoundly joined in the business of dealing with diabetes. With this comes a deep level of emotional attachment along with a vast amount of responsibility. Except for times when the challenges from diabetes necessitate putting my own needs first, my dog takes precedence, almost always.

Veterinary care, health insurance (highly recommended), training classes, equipment, safety issues, meals, behavior motivators (toys, treats, bells, clickers), exercise and human-canine bonding together create a near-constant to-do list of dog-related tasks that often override my own preferences and activities. Traveling this road has been exhilarating but definitely not insignificant.

My abounding affection for Abbey has sometimes concealed the reality of what it has taken to make this kind of animal an unconditional member of my family. Now fully trained to be my lifesaving teammate, she cannot be disregarded for long, as she has an important job to do. Accustomed to mega levels of attention, when I ignore her by focusing on my writing or studio work, or leaving home to travel, in particular, careful planning is essential. Placing her into the high-walled dog yard for long hours or days on end doesn't help her thrive; often a house sitter or nearby relative capable of relieving the stress of my absence must be called in. With the advent of the Covid-19 pandemic, sheltering at home—a wise recommendation for those living with diabetes or any other underlying medical condition—has made Abbey a very happy camper basking in the company of her pack. The pandemic's impact on my comfort level with taking her with me to the grocery store, Costco, Target, Staples and other familiar places? Not so much. Our public teaming remains on hold.

In general, however, the reaction to our teamwork and presence compels me to consider how to set boundaries and when to enforce them. There is never a time when Abbey accompanies me into a store, wearing a service vest, when I am not forced to wrestle with these issues. Questions like "May I pet your dog?" or "What kind of service dog is she?" are common. On innumerable outings, I overhear people acknowledge her working status—particularly to their children. This is reassuring that people know enough about service dogs to say "Oh, she's working, huh?" I nod and smile while trying to move on. Or: "What a sweet dog! Look at her, Jess (or Vic, or Mark, or Sara). See her working? We can't touch her right now" only to have them watch us move through the store and plead at a later "chance" encounter if I can possibly let them touch Abbey since "she's so special."

This clash in many people knowing how they should behave versus actually doing it is a complicated matter—compounded, I believe, because of the largely invisible nature of diabetes. Diabetes has no readily detectible signs of physical disability unless an emergency triggers more obvious hints like a visible insulin pump, ringing alarms, or unconcealed checks of glucose levels on a CGM or meter. I constantly discern strangers trying to add up the pieces of this puzzle to gauge why I might need to be accompanied by a service dog—perceived in the furrow of an observer's brow; the furtive but deeply inquisitive assessment given.

I've learned to shrug some of it off. To answer questions without bristling. To move quickly and purposefully when there's no extra time to give and thus discourage interactions. But the curiosity is always there, noted in people's body language that reveals their attempts to understand. Some can't help themselves—pushing past the unspoken norm of maintaining personal boundaries. One of the toughest questions I'm asked is: "Are you training her for you?" The dilemma is in how to answer these queries: how much energy or concern should I give to these encounters? My responses—whether revealing or not—plop me into a stewpot that forces me to struggle with which nuggets of truth to share.

What I've come to realize is that people's interest is natural and mostly compassionate. Profound responses aren't needed or expected; strangers are much more interested in contact with my dog—who typically wears a service coat that identifies her only as a service dog and not a DAD—than in me. Abbey's ability to draw strangers to us has eased my way in allowing some closer interactions by bending a few boundaries for the sake of my canine ambassador.

Demanding? Remarkably so. But Abbey has opened my eyes in many ways. By earning my respect through DAD skills that literally hold my fate, to some degree, in her capable brain, nose and paws, I have been willing to assume the enormous level of responsibility required for her well-being and care. In shaping my dog's behaviors and training her as a successful DAD, I accept the fact that I, alone, brought about this situation. There are days when I ask myself: *What were you thinking?*

It is then that I realize that despite the hurdles in this path, I would still follow the same one. I'd still make the same choices and do it all over again. The trek has been arduous but fun, generating challenges that included opportunities to gain resilience. The gifts of my deep relationship with Abbey, her skills designed to help me live beyond the daily challenges of diabetes, and those unexpected soulful connections with others: these have been a most glorious outcome.

My life in DAD-land continues its momentum, abounding with wonder as Abbey now works alongside me, demonstrating what she knows to our youngest canine member-in-training—puppy Ever. 'Watch me, smart puppy, and learn,' she seems to say through her actions. When my sugar levels dive, she steps in to corral the next generation with a 'Nudge. Touch. Ring the bell.'

It's all wondrous new territory to explore, so we start yet again. For me, unabashedly in love with dogs and willing to harness their innate abilities to make a difference in people's lives, this has been a wish and a promise well worth the journey.

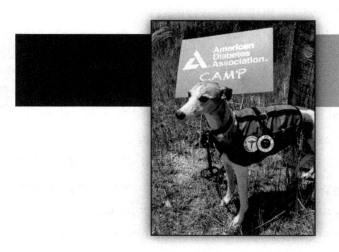

Chapter 24

Off To Camp We Go

Diabetes camp, and camp in general, has always represented an integral part of my life; one where indescribably deep relationships grow from the shared reality of living with diabetes, and being able to laugh at and lament some of the aspects that mark each person's journey. Every one of these compelling camp experiences continue to guide my life years after my first immersion just weeks after being diagnosed.

For Abbey and me, they are sure to be intensely captured within this first-ever camp session we spend together in the Manzano Mountains. While I ready Team Abbey for camp immersion, my own preparations are marked by anticipation. It will be Abbey's and my first time there for a full week, and everything that can happen is plausible. It will be my first time staying the full duration of camp in over twenty years. I am filled with dreams of connecting deeply with staff and campers and their families, but what I first have to face is more realistic and immediate: there is lots of work to be done if I am to accomplish the tasks I'd been asked to do as a volunteer and ADA Board member.

Frantically aware of the countdown to camp, I spend most mornings packing a few lidded boxes full of dog kibble, abundant treats, dishes, a blanket, leashes and a few toys. A portable red canvas crate, helpful when Abbey needs a quiet place to retreat, is wiped clean and stacked alongside a growing pile. My to-do list and ideas multiply in exponential fashion; scattered printouts mark a trail from my home office to the kitchen. In between all these preparations, I drive madly, on time stolen from essential tasks, to Abbey's final vest fitting appointment with Francie so she can finish up a lightweight service dog coat and new DAD tags. Picking them up can't be pushed back even a week. Everything seems to be a priority, crashing together in a cacophony of demands. Get ready; be ready, the Siren chants to me in rising drumbeats that pulse louder, more insistent, with each remaining day.

The final week before camp, my husband asks why I am up so late at night. Crates, two stuffed duffels, blankets, pillows, a sleeping bag and more are stacked high in the dining room along the entire length of our six-foot table.

"Didn't you have enough time to get everything done today?" His voice contains a touch of disbelief that I'm still not finished. I understand he finds it implausible that I'm not ready to step away from it all, but there's so much yet to do.

"I have to pull together an outline of what I'll actually be teaching the kids about Abbey," I insist. "A list to demonstrate what she does as a DAD and another one to get the kids more involved and try a few commands on her so they can reward her with treats. I need to make a few big signs to post too."

"All right," he says, "don't stay up too late though."

Brushing off his concern, another thought grabs me and I slip in another must-do. "Oh boy," I add. "Directions for an art activity—I almost forgot. It might be nice for the kids to make bracelets with dog charms or words with letter beads so they can take home DAD bracelets."

He stops, eyebrows arched, unable to resist asking, "Really? How important is that?"

"Oh, very, I think." My eyes avoid his, while I conjure the image that combines demonstrating DAD behaviors, getting campers to work with her and ending with the art project, until it's just perfect and makes sense. Then I meet his questioning face.

As a means of explanation, I try to share my thinking. "I can see some of these kids falling in love with Abbey, and this way, they can have a memento of their experience that supports them when they're not at camp or around her."

Bob shakes his head slightly. He knows I have my reasons for pulling together the activity. Nothing he says can easily deter me once my vision is set. I settle happily at my computer, working into the wee hours of the next morning as the printer hums away.

I pack the car early Saturday morning, wondering how I'll fit everything into the space. There's so much I've been asked to do: teach three DAD sessions, photograph camp activities and pull together a camp memory book. It's a lot to accomplish in less than six full days, and my car is stuffed nearly to the ceiling with more supplies than I'll likely use.

"Just do what you can do," Bob reminds me as I stand beside my over-packed car.

I nod. I'm nothing if not determined.

"Okay, Abster, let's go!" I call my girl, dressed in her beautiful, new, summer-weight DAD vest, to the car.

"Jump!" I command.

Then I fasten Abbey's car safety harness while silently thanking Francie for her amazing skill and effort in pulling the vest together in record time. Directions through the mountains east of Albuquerque and on to Chilili and Torreon are within reach. I double check them, roll down my window to peck my husband on the cheek and thank him for his help, and head off to the New Mexico Camp for Kids with Diabetes at Manzano Mountain Retreat.

A strange realization hits me as I'm headed to camp today: despite being grown, I still feel very much like that ten-year-old kid grappling with a life-changing first year marked by diabetes. The child who, so many decades ago, was carried in a coma into an emergency room. The child who was hospitalized for ten days in an antiseptic world where the word "diabetes" was, unbelievably, unspoken in my presence and only introduced through a nurse assigned to hand me reading material—a markedly unfunny comic book about the great tennis star Arthur Ashe who also lived with diabetes. She returned the next day with an orange, a distilled bottle of water, and a syringe for practicing drawing up and injecting the pseudo-insulin into that ridiculous piece of fruit. *Who needs this?* I'd wondered, with scant clues it was me. Secrecy abounded even at my own expense. Some details never leave you.

As I drive east, I think about how my life has been indelibly changed by living with Type 1 all these years. Heading to the New Mexico camp draws me right back to that time of youthful innocence followed by the crush of piercing torment at the unfairness of it all. So much naiveté, gone in the blink of an eye.

It was only two short months after being diagnosed that Camp Firefly entered my life. It was my parents' decision to send me there; not mine. I only recall wanting to retreat—preferring to nest and tend fresh wounds. But forced to go, it connected me with fellow peers living with diabetes for two weeks that summer and in ongoing years. It was the first time a feeling of normalcy touched my new world. It turned my views upside down by offering something I didn't know I needed: something potent and far-reaching. One where I eventually realized, in spite of what other campers and I had in common, I'd have to become a warrior of sorts to survive.

The connections made in my own first few summers at diabetes camp continue to drive me now. Who could have guessed their impact so many years later? Life with diabetes isn't ever easy, but I've had many experiences filled with joy. Somehow, as I follow the road to yet another diabetes camp, they all sing to me with lyrics themed in a sense of thankfulness. There's much to be grateful for, and today, traveling with my bestie Abbey, especially so.

As the miles from home begin to accrue, my stomach fills with butterflies at the uncertainties awaiting Abbey and me. I feel anxious about being assigned a space between occupied cabins where we'll be completely alone. And worried about what might happen if, being in an unfamiliar setting, my DAD doesn't alert or awaken me if my blood sugar drops dangerously low. But stealing a quick glance in my rearview mirror, I see Abbey happily settled and dismiss my worries to focus on her and my goal of sharing this skilled dog with others who express interest in her, knowing full well how too much thinking and fretting can sabotage the best of intentions.

I tell Abbey, "Wait until we get to camp. We'll set up our space in our cabin and then meet everyone after lunch. You are going to have so much fun."

Abbey eyes me, seemingly reassured at hearing my voice. Then she nuzzles her long snout into the turquoise throw for a snooze, oblivious to the questions of tomorrow and this next week.

Once past the dizzying curves east of Albuquerque, I break into song. It's an oldie but goodie from my time spent at Camp Firefly those few months after my diagnosis.

To the tune of the Notre Dame Fight Song:

Shots, shots for Camp Firefly, you bring the insulin, try not to cry.

Send those campers for a swim and don't let a shocky camper in (da da da).

We never stagger, we never fall.

We sober up on orange juice and all.

While our loyal staff members have headaches and pains galore (da da da da da da da).

All sorts of camp life memories flood back and trigger my recall of more songs. These feel like the fabric of my life; my core. In many ways, they are what hold me together, the weft woven with camp friendships, the warp marked by a feeling of community and not being quite so different while there. Maybe hope, too, is part of it; a framework that lets me labor, without giving up, to become a stronger and better person and push myself to live beyond diabetes.

Soon, we turn onto Ten Pines Road and wind toward camp. I stop midway in a screech of rolling dust to snap a few photos of Abbey in front of the ADA sign. The day promises to be a scorcher, so we hurry back into the air-conditioned car, creeping toward the dining hall to park and seek directions to our cabin. I want to unload and set up before jumping into the day's activities.

I walk into the nearby office. Abbey remains in the car with the windows partly open.

"Hola." I greet the two women inside. "Can you tell me where to find our Camp Director? I just got here for the week and need to unload things into Golden cabin." I give them my name and they point me to the dining hall.

A few quick directions later, I back the car down a hill and into a precipitously narrow space near our assigned cabin to begin the unloading process. It's hard work while holding onto my dog's leash. Abbey stresses quickly at the repetitive trips from car to bunkroom, and she gives up soon after I trip over her and drop an armful of items onto the ground, hopping onto the lower bunk where pillows and a sheet-covered mattress beckon her. Many trips later, the bedding and dog crate, feeding containers, my duffel and flashlights and fan, along with untold extras, are in place while Abbey watches and pants. It's not the first time I've wished she could pay me back by helping out just a little bit more. I'm tired, too, and a long day of orientation and staff training still await us.

I place Abbey's service vest on her with an apology. "Sorry, girl, I know it's hot. But this will help people recognize you for the job you do."

She acquiesces with her usual grace, as I stuff my own pockets with the typical gear donned by dog owners: poop sacks, wipes, a treat bag, bottled water and drinking cup—all for Abbey. It feels weighty but necessary.

I have one more essential task: driving down to the building by the pool area to set up materials needed for teaching campers and some of the staff about DADs. I check off my list: low blood sugar scent vials must go into the freezer, my DAD poster and handouts for the first activity teaching session on Day 2 need organizing, the poster must be taped onto a wall, seats set up in a learning circle, all the supplies brought for kiddos to test and make samples of their own glucose levels should be placed nearby. And for now, craft containers can be left on a counter. I usher Abbey into the car and drive toward the pool. I need to hustle to have any chance of grabbing lunch and being on time for Staff Orientation.

With my materials finally unloaded, I make a mental note to return later in the day to fine-tune my teaching supplies. Abbey and I jump into the car and I turn on the air conditioning full blast to cool us down, just as I realize that this is probably the last chance we'll get any air conditioning the rest of the week. Much too quickly, I pull the car into the designated staff parking area and bid it goodbye. There's a genuine wistfulness at leaving the luxury of modernity behind while Abbey and I trudge uphill on the dusty trail to the mess hall.

Wow, Abbey's very first year at diabetes camp! Everything is new to her! I remind myself to try seeing camp through her eyes. To take nothing for granted. To help her acclimate. I am momentarily dumbstruck by the cavernous "firsts" facing us. Not knowing in the least how the scenario of "a girl and her dog" will unfold, I swing open the heavy wooden door to the wood-beamed, rustic dining hall and we enter, together, into the cool darkness.

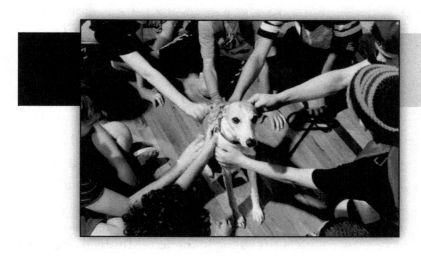

Chapter 25

Overcoming Doubters And Challengers

My first summer with Abbey at our state's American Diabetes Association camp helps me understand that while most people are open to the support provided by a DAD and embrace the confident feelings that these dogs elicit, some battles with a few people I call "doubters and challengers" are tougher. Winning, or even hoping to arrive at a draw, is often not worth the effort unless you are willing to persevere.

It's Orientation Day—the day before campers arrive for a hectic, crazy, "I-wouldn't-give-this-up-for-anything" kind of experience. I've been with the counselors and counselors-in-training (CITs) for more hot, stifling hours than all of us imagined possible.

Toward the very end of the orientation when we are all nearly at our breaking point, the Camp Director finally segues into introducing Abbey the DAD and me. I lope to the center of the gym, look around and gulp. There are no nurses and no docs from the medical staff in sight: just the same small group of young people; mostly counselors and CITs. It doesn't matter, I think—not ready to admit that it does. Fans hum in vain trying to change the humid, hot air into a cool wash.

"This is Abbey," I state. "She is my Diabetic Alert Dog—also called a Diabetes Alert Dog or DAD. Abbey is three years old and trained to signal me when my blood sugar drops below sixty-five. There are times she has alerted me to "lows" twenty minutes before my meter gives me this information. Twice, so far, she's saved my life."

I observe a few counselors nodding in interest. Mostly, though, the entire group encircling Abbey and me appears bone-weary. *How am I going to include them?*

"Who would like to come up and work with Abbey?"

That does the trick, and for the next fifteen minutes, I fly through commands with my girl as she demonstrates her magic.

"Abbey, touch."

"Abbey, nudge."

"Abbey, what is it?" I ask as I furtively reveal, tucked into my shorts pocket, a bottled sample containing a cotton pad scented with saliva from one of my low blood sugars. Abbey immediately nudges my thigh.

"Más," I tell her in Spanish. "More." She nudges me harder, and I fork over a hefty treat for her diligence. She doesn't notice me handing the scent sample vial to Sonia—a young CIT.

"Go ahead," I urge. "Ask her the same question."

"Abbey," says Sonia in a tiny, high voice, lifting her hands and arms like I just did. Before she can spit out the words, Abbey is nudging her leg, too, and the few counselors who aren't droopy-eyed murmur approval.

We wrap up our session with a quick Q & A and reach an agreement on when and how campers can approach Abbey each day. Helen, the camp director, sends the group on their way, staying behind to talk with me.

"I'm really sorry the med staff didn't come," she says. "I know you're disappointed."

"Yes," I admit. "They were busy with other things, I guess. We'll see what happens this week, okay?" I shrug and manage a tired smile.

Helen winks. "Great job," she says. "See you later." She checks her watch and runs out the gym door, heading to set up this evening's after-dinner staff activity.

Campers arrive early the next morning as we greet and send them to check in, meet with medical staff and then find their assigned cabins. A few campers seem forlorn and sidle up to Abbey. I watch them and think. *Maybe it will help if I bring Abbey into one of the cabins and try to bolster some of the more homesick and new-to-camp kiddos.* I decide to head to one of the younger boys' cabins during pre-dinner medical rounding. This is a time when physicians help campers work out their best insulin dosages to cover dinner's carbohydrates and evening activities.

"Shhh," I tell Abbey as we approach our destination, "try to be quiet."

Squeeeeak! The door hinge heaves as I tiptoe in, failing miserably at a discreet entry. Everyone bolts upright.

"Sit with me!"

"No, me!"

"Abbey, come here," begs another.

"Boys," warns a counselor who is visibly upset, "focus on what you have to do."

Two docs—one in charge and the other a resident and newcomer—are meeting with a camper and senior counselor. They look up at the commotion and quickly turn back to their task, trying to ignore us. I hear them ask how much insulin the boy needs to cover the carbs he wants to eat at dinner.

"Shhhh," I tell Abbey and nearby campers motioning us to them. "I'll come to you as you wait for your turn, but we need to be quiet now."

I know how important this time with the doctors is for each camper; how short their time is together before the dinner line forms. But what I can't gauge is whether our presence is a help or a hindrance.

"I just love her," says John. "Stay here, Abbey, please," he pleads.

We stay for two short minutes at the edge of John's bunkbed while he strokes Abbey's head. His body begins to relax and a soft hint of a smile replaces his earlier agitation as Abbey leans in.

When John is called to meet with the Rounding Team, I move with Abbey next to two more boys before the dinner bell rings. Everyone who has finished taking their meal-time insulin scrambles outside, up the hill toward the dining hall, excited about their first meal at camp and hearing the announcements for tonight's big activity.

The ax doesn't take long to fall. The next day, I pass a group of camp medical staff on the trail toward the pool as they walk together.

"Hi there," I say.

No response.

I hear a laugh. Actually, it's a snicker.

One says in a low but audible voice to the person next to him, "Why is that dog here, anyway?"

My stomach lurches. Emotions spark. I feel my internal voice rising along with anger and a growing sense of injustice. But the words stay inside me even as I think them. My heart pounds, but it's not over.

He continues, his head hanging down, wrapped in a conspiratorial huddle. What gives him away is the quick furtive movement his eyes make as he stares his challenge right at me in the seconds that we cross paths.

He sneers, "And what does that dog do, anyway?"

I want to run. To cry. Scream. Anything but do what I need to do— find the courage to directly answer his question. Instead, I say nothing. My ability to confront the matter for what it is fails me in this ill-spirited blindside.

What doesn't he understand? Why this blatant anger?

It is so harsh a challenge, so threatening, that I see only a black and white choice and nothing in between: to tuck away my wounded feelings and try to salvage our first time at the week-long camp, or to leave immediately and return home. I reluctantly choose the first option to avoid living with the aftermath of being a quitter. Somehow, I find enough strength to not give up.

Abbey and I step back from cabin visits. We connect one by one with campers and other staff willing to open themselves to getting to know us better. We give DAD training sessions that demonstrate just how smart, well-trained and vital a team we are together. I show campers how to start working with their own dogs through games and fun routines so that they, too, might think about shaping their own dogs into the same type of lifeline. I invite questions—building a basic understanding about DADs and their role in easing the burdens of this disease. Often, Abbey and I find ourselves alongside campers and staff without the need to speak at all as they reach out for a quick touch or caress. For those open to having us there as a team, these strategies work. But the bile in my throat remains while I fervently avoid any more interactions with my angry challenger.

*****

Avoidance solves nothing, of course. In the aftermath of camp and feeling so much hurt, I struggle letting go of my anger. The medical staff I most hoped would be, or could be, intelligent advocates for people and families who need a DAD, leave me shaking with disappointment. The personal impact and my sense of rejection are profound. It is a harsh, blunt lesson; you can't win them all.

My way forward is halting and takes months of deliberation. It comes from accepting what Abbey and I accomplish at camp as well as seeing that every staff member is there to make a difference. My understanding about our roles and sense of boundaries deepens, too: observing that every single one of us holds our own goals and missions dear; that we need to allow space, time and a willingness to uphold the goals and knowledge that every adult volunteer brings to our campers. That heavy feeling in my throat dissipates one unexpected winter day when I miraculously and clearly see these truths; that all Camp 180° adult volunteers have the same passion and goal of making a difference. Just as Francie tried to help me understand months ago, how quickly we tend to draw the wrong picture and conclusions when we can't step outside our own egos and frames of reference.

I return, much wiser and stronger, the next year to diabetes camp, keeping in mind the constraints each and every one of us has in our views of our impactful roles at camp. I gain new appreciation for the importance of building a village of people who don't necessarily have the same lens for how we view our work or the world. I continue to share my passion about Diabetic Alert Dogs with a smaller camp community.

Change isn't easy, but it is often good. That is evidenced by the open acceptance eventually bestowed upon not only Abbey but yet another nurse-owned DAD team who joins the camp medical staff. This is a summer with lots of laughter embraced by everyone at camp— including my earlier challenger. With this, healing comes.

A few months post-camp, I am privileged to attend a graduation ceremony held by Assistance Dogs of the West (ADW). This talented group is based in Santa Fe, New Mexico. They engage dozens of school children, veterans and individuals in court-ordered diversion programs in the training of their service dogs. Their job is to raise and love these Labrador retrievers, expose them to a multitude of sights, sounds and experiences and polish their enormous desire to please and learn new tasks, thus nurturing every canine personality.

It takes anywhere from a year to two years to socialize each pup while professional trainers decide what specialized jobs each dog can best do to provide a life-changing partnership with their human match. Love and respect are the warp to the weave of socialization and training. The thread that binds all this devoted work is the belief that every person's life can be better; that we all deserve an ally to fill in where there are weaknesses or losses, forming a happier, more fulfilled existence through the uniqueness of the human-canine bond.

In the James A. Little Theater at the New Mexico School for the Deaf, there are no more than a handful of empty seats as the graduation ceremony begins. I observe the audience audibly trilling with excitement and place myself against the back wall in order to take it all in. It is then, in the sudden hush of hundreds of voices, that I glimpse actress Ali MacGraw stepping from a far aisle onto the stage—carrying a wriggling yellow Lab pup—to introduce the teams and their graduating service dogs. Her presence stuns in its regal simplicity: she has long pulled-back dark hair streaked in silver, understated clothing and a genuine smile lighting her face. But it is her words and commitment to the mission of ADW that resonate:

"Welcome to the Assistance Dogs of the West 2017 graduation." Ms. MacGraw hands the squirming puppy to a nearby assistant while we ooh and aww at the precious bundle and lean in to hear more.

"ADW's founders, trainers and volunteers do some of the most important work that can be done, and it is through this call to action that I believe we can make a difference in our communities and the very challenging world confronting us today. Let love change your world."

And with that, my heart opens: to the stories about the courthouse facility dogs—trained to stand with elders, children and other victims of violence while they find the courage to tell their stories in San Francisco, Los Angeles, Tulare County and Austin; and to the searing tale of a young girl brought into the Children's Advocacy Center and CASA in Chavez County, New Mexico, so broken by a lifetime of violent sexual assaults that she couldn't speak a word until she touched Ben, an enormous chocolate Lab. Only then did she share the harrowing details of what she had endured by sobbing and whispering into his ear as he provided her with warmth and safety.

My heart embraces two owner-handlers who participated in ADW's Owner/Self Training of their own service dogs—much like my own training of Abbey—and found themselves able to push away loneliness, fear and a sense of defeat at their physical challenges with the support of their canine companions. If it takes a village to create and power change, these compassionate stories shared by volunteers only sweeten the invitation.

Belief. Love. Forgiveness. Friendship. Hope. Joy. I try to live these words in the fullest sense—all enhanced by training and having a DAD. Abbey makes my life richer than I ever thought possible. A few goals that once seemed impossible are within reach. She has gifted me with a deep level of confidence, helped me believe in myself and moved me to take a more conscious, active role in managing my day-to-day health. Mine is a significant testament, consistently supported by similar accolades shared by each person whose life has been touched by service dogs and DADs.

My mission is much like ADW's—to take up the banner for opening people's eyes to the benefits of Diabetic Alert Dogs for those who need and want them in spite of resistance expressed from doubters and challengers. Having the opportunity to own and share my DAD with others helps me make a difference by offering guidance and supporting training, particularly as the rates of diabetes soar worldwide. With about 10.5 percent of the U.S. population (34.2 million), alone, currently diagnosed with diabetes (National Diabetes Statistics Report 2020), we have to do something more as the costs and toll of diabetes continue to skyrocket. Advocating for the security and companionship that a DAD can bring to people's lives is a viable option; a beautiful and important antidote to the isolation and fears brought on by this long-term health challenge in a difficult world.

And what of the doubters and challengers? What can be said of the arguments and motives behind some of the conflicts?

Investigating underlying issues faced by many people living with diabetes reveals why the clamoring at camp over Abbey even exists, by recognizing that the desire to hold, touch and reach out for these dogs is a helpful, effective method for breaking down feelings of isolation and difference. Any quality of life survey proves this. For now, most of what we have are anecdotal reports, though there are a growing number of scientific studies that support people who live with or have trained Medical Detection or Medical Assistance Dogs lead happier lives.

Fighting these findings and preferring to place trust in technology over bestowing belief in a dog—even one that is presumably trained with specific alerting skills—is the norm among clinicians. Medical personnel tend to recommend what they know and trust, and the honest truth is that most know very little about the high standards to which DADs are trained. It is a rare physician or diabetes educator who has time to investigate the training process or its benefits.

I grasp the dilemma: there is a sense of discomfort in endorsing the role of a Diabetes Alert Dog in patients' lives because the impact *seems* unscientific, is difficult to measure and clinical training makes it easier to recommend medical technologies based on science. But while this thinking appears to have rational roots, technology is not infallible in terms of financial, physical and emotional costs. A well-trained dog that alerts to high and/or low glucose is an exquisite back-up tool in the diabetes management kit. Every one of these tools—including the trained DAD—has a measurable impact and is capable, either singly or in combination, of changing lives for the better.

There is yet one more side to consider when thinking about doubters and challengers; the view that recognizes that *having a DAD is transformational.* It is a story of magic—one of rekindled hope, deeply abiding companionship and an antidote to worries that accompany diabetes; a sweet dance between partners that is based on gratitude and joy. Those of us lucky enough to have these dogs describe markedly less diabetes stress, a deeper belief in ourselves, acknowledgement of the gifts provided by DADs and a drive to use the profound level of satisfaction we get from our DADs to pay the gift forward by giving back to our communities.

It is truly as simple as this: nothing is more emotionally supportive and life-altering than a devoted dog trained to be your helper, partner and dependable friend. Teamed with new technologies, a DAD is capable of backing these diabetes management tools to create the most exquisite "total package" for the best possible outcomes.

For me, knowing the benefits, I stand squarely on the side of "arming" people with one of the most joyous tools I've found in a lifetime of battling and actively managing diabetes. I own my life now: diabetes doesn't own or define me. My journey has been long and intense, but empowering and worthwhile. I have finally emerged and become a warrior of the sweetest kind—one where I have learned how to let love and my DAD's incredible skills change my world.

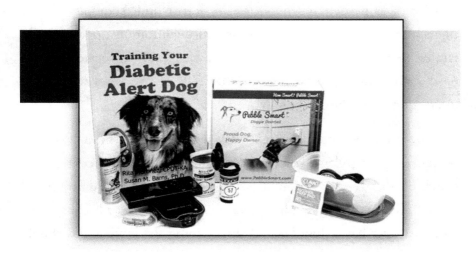

Chapter 26

General Recommendations

I f you think that having a Diabetes/Diabetic Alert Dog can help you or someone you love, then you owe it to yourself to give it serious consideration. Used in collaboration with other diabetes management tools, a trained DAD becomes part glucose alert-indicator (great for when new CGM sensors are counting down to their official startup) and an empowering emotional support specialist that moves people with diabetes into an active decision-making role. Once you decide this choice is viable, there are more questions and issues to tackle before determining a course of action.

One critical first step is to read the Federal laws and statutes for the Americans with Disabilities Act (ADA) that guarantee your right to be accompanied by a canine specifically-trained to assist those with medical conditions, as needed, in public places. If you are raising a child living with diabetes, consider whether a Section 504 Plan (referred to as "a

504 Plan") is needed at school, too. A deeper understanding of your rights after assessing your own needs and qualifications, or those of a family member, will help you more knowledgeably advocate for your needs, albeit in the most upbeat and collaborative ways to sweeten interactions with those around you.

There are a wealth of organizations and dog trainers available. Ask people attending classes in your neighborhood training centers and search on the web for possibilities. You'll find many you didn't know existed. Groups and individuals receiving praise are worth contacting. The best ones have often been at this training the longest and should have a great record of success. Use a checklist to ask questions when you talk with representatives or trainers. I trust a number of them, but it pays to talk to graduates of programs, other self-trainers and buyers. It is just as critical to maintain a deep level of personal commitment for continued training once you get a DAD from any of these groups or individuals.

The problem I faced, and one that may confront you, too, is the proverbial elephant in the room. How much can you afford to pay to train a Diabetes/Diabetic Alert Dog? The first step is to figure out the cost difference between getting a fully-trained DAD or training your own dog to have these skills. Whatever you choose, you still need to do double duty by ensuring the training will work for you and your diabetes (or that of a family member). You will need to visit, ask questions and gain skills in interacting in specific ways with your promised DAD.

Training takes a lot of time, and you should prepare for a minimum commitment of one year. It is often longer with an average training span of eighteen months to two years for a dog and handler to learn basic service dog and alerting behaviors, as well as socialization and safety commands for going into public places. As time equals money, you can appreciate that having someone else train your intended DAD will, by necessity, add up to a certain, generally high, cost.

Some of these costs may be partially underwritten by an endocrinologist's statement of need based on volumes of data as well as your insurance coverage. Increased media coverage and online advertising for dogs trained by businesses specifically for those in need is raising the demand for such valuable animals. This has given rise to the possibility of applying for grants or scholarships from various groups advertising on the internet, although scams have also increased. You may find a number of funders that support your efforts to obtain a DAD. Be curious but cautious about large, up-front financial commitments. Ask questions and be open to possibilities. You have nothing to lose.

One essential point for those able to afford and purchase already-trained Diabetic Alert Dogs is recognizing that additional in-home and ongoing training to become an effective team must be a long-term commitment. A DAD team becomes more effective with consistent, personalized training, even if your dog has already been trained by someone else. Knowing this will offset disappointment when your "ready-trained" DAD does not perform in the ways you need and expect. Active teaching and ongoing interactions in your own home with your key team members will make the difference between success and failure.

If you can't afford a ready-trained DAD but can fully commit to working with an established dog trainer or group who can support you with the process, detail by detail and task by task, then you might very well consider training your own dog. This plan is more affordable for most people than choosing a dog trained by an outside organization. That is, IF your dog has the right temperament. IF s/he has acceptable public behaviors. IF s/he … you get the idea. There are published resources and, best of all, good rates of success for owner-trained DADs. My own two dogs fall into this last group, and they are a huge asset to my own diabetes management.

Just as crucial is your commitment as the trainer. These criteria for determining the trainability of dogs as DADs apply equally to you. Ask yourself: Do I have enough time, adequate patience and willingness to perform due diligence by reading and structuring DAD training? Can I afford to pay a local canine trainer-mentor, work together, and promise enough patience to commit to building each and every step of the needed training? There are a multitude of "ifs" to contemplate in the process of training your own DAD, and each one is essential to address honestly and completely.

Teaching your own DAD or service dog isn't for everyone. In fact, it's a very difficult task to accomplish. I asked myself these questions, too, and then sought out another trainer capable of assessing my dog. Fortunately, she found my first to-be-trained dog Abbey to have ample intelligence, owner-attentiveness and a non-flappable temperament. Once we got her "okay" on trainability, she asked me to reflect deeply, over many weeks, on these questions: "Do I need a DAD?" and "How will I feel about being reminded about my diabetes 24/7?" before beginning our formal training program.

One fact is clear: There is no going back once you commit to the training of a DAD. Your dog, with your support, will have a vital job to enact the rest of his or her life. You must be willing to pledge yourself to nurturing the best in both of you. If you can do this and understand the necessity of conducting ongoing training sessions, then the world of shaping your own DAD is probably like a very seductive treat tempting you to connect with all the fun, camaraderie and canine support that you dream of.

Whether you build your own DAD team, like I did, or you decide to find a dog trained by others through different means, your life will be enriched, your days filled with more joy, and your nights wrapped in hope and diminished fears. The depth of the human-canine bond is all-empowering and inspirational; it's a relationship to marvel and an invitation to live more fully in the here and now. For me, it decreases my feelings of isolation and keeps me on track—active and in love with the gift of life—every single day. Nothing much else matters. For those of us with diabetes, and for those who love us, it is nearly everything.

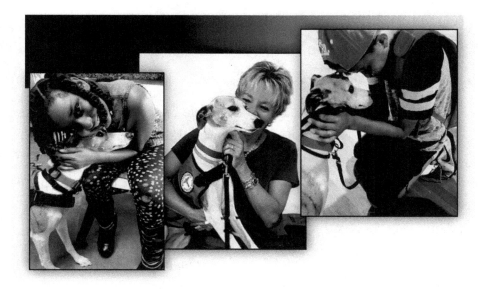

Chapter 27

The Age Of Wisdom

Not so very long ago, an interaction with yet another complete stranger brought home the incredible power of the human-dog relationship. It has both nothing and everything to do with Abbey's role as my DAD.

"Hey, Abbey," I say, "let's run into Wal-Mart and pick up a few things."

I freely admit that I talk to my best friend and 24/7 source of support all the time. Today is no different as my ever-observant companion seems to listen and concur while I park the car.

We enter the open doors, garnering smiles and nods from many shoppers. Determined not to dally, I move forward a few feet to my first stop and peruse the shelves for hair items after giving Abbey a firm "stay" command.

Be focused. Don't waste any time.

But just an arm's length away, I can't help but note that a woman is staring at us. She seems to send out a powerful signal that beseeches my attention and doesn't stop. Perhaps it is Abbey's impeccable behavior? I sigh and turn, realizing that something must give; that I need to open myself to what I hope will be a short exchange with yet another someone I don't really know.

She moves closer and says, "I just love your dog. She reminds me of my most special dog that I lost. She was my life."

I'd begun stepping away but am now anchored to my spot.

"Such an empty hole in my life, even when I think of her now. She still touches me. Like your sweet girl."

"Well," I suggest gently, "maybe it's time to get another dog to fill your heart?"

"Oh," she tells me, "I have two dogs and two cats. This special dog left us years ago but I still cry when I think about her."

My throat constricts. I nod as waves of hurt and empathy wash over me. We'd just put down our eldest girl two weeks ago. It has only been in the last few days that I haven't sobbed, thinking of my sweet Zoe Rose, all the while feeling so thankful for my heart dog beside me.

I move closer to this stranger just as she steps toward Abbey and me. We seem to be drawn together through some inexplicable force. It's a pulse of emotion for me—almost overwhelming in its power and the unanticipated connection between the two of us.

"I've often wondered," I confide, "why we're so hurt when our pets leave us. I think it's because they are such a deep part of us, and everything we feel and live through is marked by their presence."

She nods with tears in her eyes.

I muse, "When they go, it's like this trusted witness to our lives, our feelings, just vanishes. My world felt empty when I lost my Zoe."

"Oh," she says, "I'm so sorry. So much love you had for her."

I agree by lowering my head as my eyes draw tears at these raw truths. Somehow, the experience of loving and learning and being changed by our treasured dogs has moved us from complete strangers into something else I can't quite define. The feeling and pull are palpable—extraordinarily intense.

She continues, "I believe, like my father told me before he left this life, that all the animals we hold dear will meet us. My father said, 'Look for me by a bridge surrounded by the dogs. You'll find me there.'"

The lump in my throat swells.

We both know the value of that devotion. We have both been touched by it—changed by it. All I can do is stare into the eyes of this beautiful stranger and reach out to hug her. No more words pass between us. None are needed.

I remember my wise friend Ramona recently saying, "Think of all the things we've learned and how it's bringing us into the age of wisdom." And my friend Francie's mantra to "live in gratitude." These words can't help but propel my thinking about my experiences and the understandings I've gained due to managing diabetes all these years: the touch of profound friendships; the gratitude of being able to travel; the years spent shaping lives through teaching; the utter joy of building a family through adoption; the literal lows of crashing blood sugars; the interminable waits for life to recalibrate to normal after soaring glucose episodes; the pesky and all-too-humbling ER visits; the fears and the what-ifs—there are so many; the immeasurable time spent training my first DAD. All of it only matters because the journey has brought me here. This woman's connection to her dog, just like mine, brings me to my knees in appreciation of my life, its lessons and gifts and my beautiful canine soulmate and friend.

With Abbey's help to live more readily with my diabetes, I am that much stronger and steadier. It helps to share her focus on living completely in the here and now. Watching her leap into spirited, joyful play becomes my joy, my path. With her distinct alerting skills and gift of unconditional love, I am filled with gratitude and purpose.

As someone who long wanted to run away from the burdens of diabetes, my life is fuller now. Easier. I can smile at the gift of my beloved Diabetic Alert Dog and remind myself that this is not such a bad place to be.

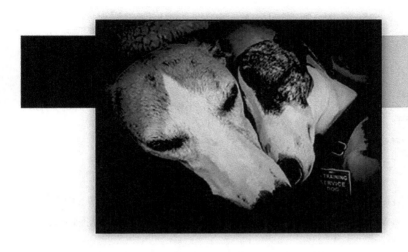

Afterword

The more I get out into the community with my Diabetes/Diabetic Alert Dogs, the more I connect with people who are deeply impacted by this disease. They clamor for the type of support that Abbey and Ever represent as unofficial DAD ambassadors. I hope that sharing my DADs' skills in diverse community settings inspires a new generation of Diabetes/Diabetic Alert Dog teams so that the toll of diabetes stress and isolation is markedly transformed. Abbey, Ever and I would love to hear from you! Reach us for support and information at *SugarBark.net.*

Acknowledgments

Deepest thanks to those who have helped me reach my goal of becoming a working Diabetes/Diabetic Alert Dog team. Thank you for reminding me that despite the greatest challenges we face, whether health-based or other, there is no discounting the power of a fellow human or animal's love in transforming one's life.

Leslie Jordan, of Artistry Whippets, for gifting me with my precious, remarkably capable, wily DAD companions Gabby Abbey and Ever.

Canine trainer Arie Deller for your mentoring and sustained belief that Abbey and I would succeed in our unusual quest.

Extraordinary vet Dr. Consuela Conley and fellow NM Lobo Lure Coursing Club friends; thank you for opening my eyes to everything hounds and these breeds can be.

Frances Zeller for your sage advice, insights, love and zany laughter.

Fellow writers Kristina Caffrey, Karen Glinski, Catherine Harding-Adams, Evelynn Moore and Desiree Perriguey for pushing me onward through chapters thick and thin.

Photographer Cheryl Cathcart of Cheryl Cathcart Photography for so beautifully capturing Abbey's spirit so that it can be shared with others.

Pat and Barbara Carr of Carr Imaging for your substantial role in helping these photographs for the book come to solid fruition.

Julie McVay, my soul sister, inspiration and touchstone, who lives life with gratitude and a gracious belief in all things good while challenging the impact of this long-term disease.

Helen Pappas, colleague and longtime friend, for painting my dreams and life with hope.

Fellow ADA Community Leadership Board members, community health activists, ADA-NM Camp 180° Committee, staff, campers and families, JDRF compatriots, Type 1 Divas, Dr. George King and Joslin 50 Year Medalists for the joy inspired by our mutual journey and your unmatched passion to make a difference.

And finally, to my husband Bob, whose motto it is to always move forward toward "making it so!" Your positive outlook lights my way, and that is everything.

Diabetes/Diabetic Alert Dog Resources

Dogs and Specialized Scent Training Capabilities

Hahn, Lucinda. February 2020. "This dog could save your life." Southwest: The Magazine, 44-53.
Dallas: https://issuu.com/southwestmag/docs/february2020/s/10216058

American Kennel Club, How to Teach Your Dog Scent Work at Home by Kathy Santo, May 27, 2020:
https://www.akc.org/expert-advice/training/how-to-teach-your-dog-scent-work/

American Kennel Club, Why Not Give AKC Scent Work a Try? by Stephanie Gibeault, MSc, CPDT, Jan 15, 2019:
https://www.akc.org/expert-advice/lifestyle/why-not-give-akc-scent-work-a-try/

Maria Goodavage, Doctor Dogs: How our good friends are becoming our best medicine, Dutton, October 2019:
https://www.penguinrandomhouse.com/books/566960/doctor-dogs-by-maria-goodavage/9781524743048/

Diabetes Alert Dog Resources

General Information about Service-Assistance Dogs

Assistance Dogs International (member programs: Looking for an Assistance Dog)
https://assistancedogsinternational.org/main/looking-for-an-assistance-dog/

On-Line Discussion Group with Information on Service Dogs.
http://groups.msn.com/AssistanceDogs
http://groups.yahoo.com/group/exploring_service_dogs

http://herizenfyre-ivil.tripod.com/helperdogs/id3.html

Temperament Assessment & Evaluation

(general and/or for service dogs)

AKC Temperament Test, American Kennel Club:
https://www.akc.org/akctemptest/

Canine Behavioral Assessment & Research Questionnaire (C-BARQ) Evaluation, 2020, by James A. Serpell and The University of Pennsylvania, PennVet, University of Pennsylvania's Center for Interaction of Animals & Society, 2020:
https://vetapps.vet.upenn.edu/cbarq/

Psychiatric Service Dog Partners: Dogs Saving Lives, How to Pick a Adult Service Dog Prospect by Tracey Martin:
https://www.psychdogpartners.org/resources/getting-a-dog/pick-adult-service-dog-prospect

Psychiatric Service Dog Partners: Dogs Saving Lives, How to pick a service dog puppy prospect by Tracey Martin:
https://www.psychdogpartners.org/resources/getting-a-dog/pick-puppy-service-dog-prospect

Finding Diabetic Alert Dogs

(also called Diabetes Alert Dogs or DADs)

American Kennel Club, Calling 911 Canine-Style: How One Teen Found Her Diabetic Alert Dog by Elaine Waldorf Gewirtz, Feb 20, 2020: https://www.akc.org/expert-advice/training/calling-911-canine-style/

Assistance Dogs International:

http://www.assistancedogsinternational.org/membershipdirectory.php or
https://assistancedogsinternational.org/main/looking-for-an-assistance-dog/

Assistance Dogs of the West, assistancedogsofthewest.org, 505-986-9748 or 866-986-3489 (toll free), Santa Fe, NM

Dogs4Diabetics, Concord, CA, 925.246.5785 | info@dogs4diabetics.com
: https://dogs4diabetics.com/programs/dog-training/

Tattle Tail Scent Dogs, KC Owens, Salt Lake City, UT:
http://www.tattletailscentdogs.com/

Finding a reputable DAD program

Owner training of a DAD vs. program-trained DADS:
http://www.clickincanines.com/site/choose.html

Locating a reputable Canine Trainer

Certification Council for Professional Dog Trainers:
http://www.ccpdt.org/

Minimum standards for Assistance Dogs in Public Settings

Assistance Dogs International Standards:
http://www.assistancedogsinternational.org/Standards/
and https://assistancedogsinternational.org/standards/summary-of-standards/

Assistance Dogs International 'Public Access Test':
http://www.assistancedogsinternational.org/publicaccesstest.php or
www.assistancedogsinternational.org

C-BARQ Evaluation:
http://vetapps.vet.upenn.edu/cbarq/

IAADP Minimum Training Standards for Public Access, International Association of Assistance Dogs Partners (IIADP): https://www.iaadp.org/iaadp-minimum-training-standards-for-public-access.html

On Obtaining Trained Diabetes Alert Dogs/Diabetic Alert Dogs

Assistance Dogs of the West, assistancedogsofthewest.org, 505-986-9748 or 866-986-3489 (toll free), Santa Fe, NM: https://assistancedogsofthewest.org/

Dogs4Diabetics, Concord, CA, 925.246.5785 | info@dogs4diabetics.com : https://dogs4diabetics.com/programs/dog-training/

Training Your Own Diabetes/Diabetic Alert Dog (DAD)

Assistance Dogs of the West, assistancedogsofthewest.org, 505-986-9748 or 866-986-3489 (toll free), Santa Fe, NM: https://assistancedogsofthewest.org/our-programs/owner-self-training/

Rockaway, Libby, M.D. Dogs workbook: A guide to self-training your own Diabetic Alert Dog, 2018: MDDogsInc@gmail.com or http://www.mddogs.org/wp-content/uploads/2018/06/MDDogs-FINAL1- ilovepdf-compressed.pdf

Service Dogs of New Mexico (SDNM), sdnm@gmail.com, 505-274-5048 or 505-358-1366, Albuquerque, NM

SugarBark: Diabetic Alert Dog services: https://www.sugarbark.net/Tattle Tail Scent Dogs, KC Owens, Salt Lake City, UT: http://www.tattletailscentdogs.com/ http://www.tattletailscentdogs.com/

On training for retrieval of supplies or human help when alerting to blood glucose issues

Shirley's Retrieve

http://shirleychong.com/keepers/retrieve.html

Recordable dog doorbell: Bow Wow Button (two-pack):

https://www.amazon.ca/Bow-Wow-Button-

PoochieBells at onlyanocean.net. 843-380-4042:

https://onlyanocean.net/

Pebble Smart Doggie Doorbell (Keith Jin) at https://pebblesmart.com

Pet-2-Ring (Inthecompanyofdogs) at www.pet2ring.com

Training your Diabetic Alert Dog by Rita Martinez, CPDT-KA and Susan M. Barns, Ph.D., 2013; eBook: ISBN-10: 098885080X ISBN-13: 978-0-9888508-0-4; Print book: ISBN-109: 0988850818 ISBN-13: 978-0-9888508-1-1

Legal statutes

Americans with Disabilities Act (ADA) of 1990 (42 U.S.C. § 12101):

https://www.ada.gov/pubs/adastatute08.pdf

Section 504 of the Rehabilitation Act of 1973, Office for Civil Rights, Protecting students with disabilities:

https://www2.ed.gov/about/offices/list/ocr/504faq.html#:~:text=STUDENTS%20PROTECTED%20UNDER%20SECTION%20504&text=Section%20504%20requires%20that%20school,or%20more%20major%20life%20activities.

Your Legal Disability Rights: https://www.usa.gov/disability-rights and https://www.usa.gov/disability-rights#item-35762

ADA 2010 revised requirements: Service Animals

ADA Legal Brief: Service animals and individuals with disabilities under the Americans with Disabilities Act (ADA), adata.org, ADA Knowledge, Translation Center Legal Brief No. 2.1 by Sharon E. Brown, ADA Knowledge Translation Center, 2019:
https://adata.org/legal_brief/legal-brief-service-animals-and-individuals-disabilities-under-americans
disabilities#:~:text=Although%20the%20use%20of%20assistance,services%20covered%20by%20the%20ADA.

Travel with a Diabetes/Diabetic Alert Dog

Federal government may tighten restrictions on service animals on planes by Merrit Kennedy. January 23, 2020. NPR:
https://www.npr.org/2020/01/23/798662547/federal-government-may-tighten-restrictions-on-service-animals-on-planes

U.S. Department of Transportation seeks comment on proposed amendments to regulation of service animals on flights.
https://www.transportation.gov . January 22, 2020. U/S. Department of Transportation, Washington, DC 20590

About The Author

Kat Richter-Sand, Ed.D, is a 50-year Joslin Medalist and 50-year recipient of the Lily Diabetes Journey Awards, Board member of the New Mexico Affiliate of the American Diabetes Association, diabetes camp advocate, fundraiser, educator-trainer, artist and writer. Living decades with Type 1, she seeks to transform the ups and downs of this disease by connecting with others challenged by diabetes distress, 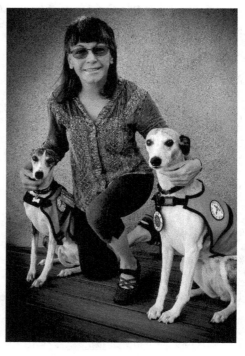 management and quality of life issues. She believes that cultivating your best self and a meaningful life come from doing what you love and learning to love what you do. Her own passions include clay, gardening, photography, travel, and training her beloved dogs, two of whom are DADs. Kat offers insights on living well with diabetes and shares the goals and methods for training these canines and the joy and peace of mind that come from teaming with Diabetes Alert Dogs. She lives in sunny Albuquerque, New Mexico and can be reached at https://www.sugarbark.net/.

About The Photographer

Cheryl Cathcart is an avid animal and nature photographer. She retired from a Research Financial VP post at Cedars-Sinai Medical Center to pursue her love of travel and art. She has traveled to many countries on all seven continents to photograph nature and animals both domestic and wild. Growing up in Wyoming, her earliest memories tap family trips to both Yellowstone and the 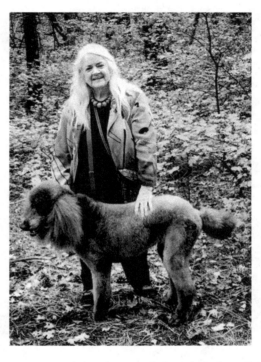 Iowa farms of her grandparents. Her work has been exhibited at the NM Farm and Ranch Historical Museum in Las Cruces, NM and the Art Museum of Southeast Texas, Gallery with a Cause at the NM Cancer Center, and local and state photography exhibitions. Cheryl lives in Corrales, NM. More of her images can be found at www.cherylcathcart.com.

CPSIA information can be obtained
at www.ICGtesting.com
Printed in the USA
LVHW050759010621
689026LV00012B/1703